Electronically Controlled Drug Delivery

Electronically Controlled Drug Delivery

Edited by

Bret Berner, Ph.D.
Cygnus, Inc.
Redwood City, California

and

Steven M. Dinh, Sc.D.
Novartis Corporation
Suffern, New York

CRC Press

Boca Raton   Boston   London   New York   Washington, D.C.

Acquiring Editor:	Liz Covello
Project Editor:	Andrea Demby
Marketing Manager:	Becky McEldowney
Cover design:	Denise Craig
PrePress:	Carlos Esser
Manufacturing:	Carol Royal

Library of Congress Cataloging-in-Publication Data

Electronically controlled drug delivery / edited by Bret Berner,
    Steven M. Dinh.
            p.   cm.
        Includes bibliographical references and index.
        ISBN 0-8493-7681-5 (alk. paper)
        1. Drug delivery systems.   2. Drug infusion pumps.   I. Berner,
    Bret.   II. Dinh, Steven M.
        [DNLM: 1. Infusion Pumps, Implantable.   2. Drug Delivery Systems-
    -methods.   3. Technology, Pharmaceutical--methods.   WB 354 E38
    1998]
    RS199.5.E43   1998
    615'.6--dc21
    DNLM/DLC
    for Library of Congress   98-15824
                                                                                    CIP

Preface

Electronically controlled drug delivery is in its infancy in terms of commercial practice and potential. While several infusion pumps are marketed for selected therapies, inconvenience for the patient is still a limiting factor. A combination of breakthroughs in microelectronics, micromachining, miniaturized analytical systems, and chronopharmacology could allow for the application of electronically controlled drug delivery to a wider range of therapies and for substantial improvements in the quality of life for these patients.

As this book goes to press, MiniMed has announced filing a 510K for its implantable glucose sensor for diabetics. This should open the door to short- and long-term trend analysis, and the ability to conduct clinical trials to determine optimal regimens to use to program implantable pumps for insulin. In a next generation product, feedback systems for drug delivery should become a reality for implantable pumps.

A number of noninvasive approaches to controlled drug delivery, in particular, iontophoresis and phonophoresis, have products in late clinical development. An iontophoretic combination product for lidocaine and epinephrine is approved and marketed. However, the difficulties of making products sufficiently robust to conduct large-scale clinical trials and for home use have extended the introduction of these noninvasive products far beyond the date that many believed. The hypothesized advantages in patient compliance and cost should make the wait worthwhile.

With programmable drug delivery becoming a reality, there is still no single text devoted to this subject. This book provides, in a single volume, chapters with (a) overviews of the fundamentals of the technologies and the therapeutic needs, (b) specific commercial applications, and (c) reviews of newer technologies. Obviously, in this rapidly expanding field, several omissions have occurred due to the time since conception of this book in 1994. Nevertheless, we hope that this compilation of technologies into a single text provides the needed stimulus to both graduate students and practicing scientists to expedite innovation in these fields.

Finally, we thank the authors for their cooperation and the quality of their contributions.

Bret Berner, Ph.D.
Steven M. Dinh, Sc.D.

The Editors

Bret Berner, Ph.D., is Vice President of Development and Analytical Sciences at Cygnus, Inc. and is currently trying to commercialize a noninvasive iontophoretic glucose monitory system. After studying physical chemistry and neurosciences, Dr. Berner received his Ph.D. from UCLA in 1978. Before joining Cygnus, Dr. Berner was Director of Basic Pharmaceutics Research at Ciba-Geigy for ten years. He has also held the positions of Director of Research at the Hercon Division of Health-Chem Corporation and as a staff scientist with The Procter & Gamble Company.

Dr. Berner is the author of over 80 patents and articles in the fields of controlled-release drug delivery and biomedical devices. He was a co-editor of the three volume series, *The Transdermal Delivery of Drugs,* also published by CRC Press.

Steven M. Dinh, Sc.D., is currently Head of Transdermals Pharmaceutical Research and Development. This unit serves Novartis Pharmaceuticals Corporation's global transdermal activities. As part of his functional responsibilities, he continues to be involved in analyzing and recommending opportunities for strategic alliances.

Dr. Dinh earned his B.E. from Cooper Union in 1976, an M.S. from Cornell University in 1978, and a Sc.D. from the Massachusetts Institute of Technology (MIT) in 1981. He then joined UCLA as an Assistant Professor in the Engineering School.

In 1982, he moved to the Pioneering Research Laboratory of DuPont, where he began his industrial career in learning how to apply basic technologies in the development of high performance materials and engineering processes. In 1987, he joined the Basic Pharmaceutics Research department at Ciba-Geigy to build the Drug Delivery Systems Development group and to pursue fundamental and applied research in novel drug delivery. He also maintains an active interest in basic research and is supervising graduate research at the Georgia Institute of Technology.

Contributors

Smita Amin, M.D.
Department of Dermatology
Toronto Hospital
University of Toronto
Toronto, Ontario, Canada

Bret Berner, Ph.D.
Cygnus, Inc.
Redwood City, California

Ronald R. Burnette, Ph.D.
School of Pharmacy
University of Wisconsin
Madison, Wisconsin

M. Begoña Delgado-Charro, Ph.D.
Centre Interuniversitaire de Recherche
  et d'Enseignement
"Pharmapeptides"
Campus Universitaire
Archamps, France

Steven M. Dinh, Sc.D.
Novartis Pharmaceuticals Corporation
Suffern, New York

Richard H. Guy, Ph.D.
Centre Interuniversitaire de Recherche
  et d'Enseignement
"Pharmapeptides"
Campus Universitaire
Archamps, France

Kenneth T. Heruth, Ph.D.
Medtronic, Inc.
Minneapolis, Minnesota

William J. M. Hrushesky, M.D.
Stratton Veterans Administration
  Medical Center
Albany, New York

Joseph Kost, Sc.D.
Department of Chemical Engineering
Ben-Gurion University
Beer-Sheva, Israel

Howard I. Maibach, M.D.
Department of Dermatology
University of California School of
  Medicine, San Francisco
San Francisco, California

Russell O. Potts, Ph.D.
Cygnus, Inc.
Redwood California

Mark R. Prausnitz, Sc.D.
School of Chemical Engineering
Georgia Institute of Technology
Atlanta, Georgia

Jagdish Singh, Ph.D.
Department of Pharmaceutical Sciences
College of Pharmacy
North Dakota State University
Fargo, North Dakota

Janet A. Tamada, Ph.D.
Cygnus, Inc.
Redwood City, California

Sietse Wouters, Ph.D.
Xemics
Neuchâtel, Switzerland

Table of Contents

Section I
Introduction

1 Electronically Assisted Drug Delivery: An Overview

Bret Berner and Steven M. Dinh

CONTENTS

1.1 INTRODUCTION

The combination of developments in microelectronics, micromachining, and medical device design, along with a recognition of the potential needs for chronotherapy, and the development of bioanalytical tools to perform the measurements has allowed the creation of a variety of electronically assisted drug delivery technologies, in particular, iontophoresis, infusion pumps, and sonophoresis. Circadian variation in the safety profile of anticancer drug therapy,[1,2] tolerance to CNS medications, the need for patient-controlled input, and the emergence of peptidic drugs that are currently practically administered as parenterals are the opportunities for these new systems. Concurrently, the development of inexpensive biosensors for home use diagnostics and the trend toward outpatient care can ultimately provide the setting for intelligent systems with feedback control.

While this vision of electronically assisted intelligent therapeutic systems is enticing, one must not forget the realities of commercial medicine. The costs of therapeutic development and distribution have escalated because of potential product liability issues and the resulting increased regulatory requirements. To provide sufficient financial returns under the burden of these costs, the threshold market size for pharmaceutical product development, other than simple line extensions, has reached hundreds of millions of dollars in sales. This has precipitated the globalization of pharmaceutical markets, harmonization of the regulatory environment, "megamergers" in the pharmaceutical industry, and the "outsourcing" of R&D to

0-8493-7681-5/98/$0.00+$.50
© 1998 by CRC Press LLC

small "boutique" companies. Medical devices have not yet reached this stage, but the same trend may be emerging.

These realities have slowed the development of electronically controlled drug delivery systems. Nevertheless, a new iontophoretic product for coadministration of lidocaine and epinephrine has been approved by the FDA and launched recently. While niche institutional therapies, involving trained nurses and patients with restricted activities, would be the logical first step in developing such systems, the required profitable market size does not permit this path. Consequently, home use therapies are the initial targets for product development and all the required "bells-and-whistles" must be included in the first generation of electronically controlled products. In particular, an iontophoretic delivery system for fentanyl is entering Phase III after several years. In addition, a disposable iontophoretic delivery system for hydromorphone is entering clinical trials. While an institutional device to replace patient-controlled analgesia would have been a more logical initial product, a home use product requires consideration of such issues as interference from static electricity caused by walking across a room or from shorting circuits by splashing.

The objective of this book is to provide an overview of advances in drug delivery to optimize therapy using electronics to regulate the delivery profile. This book is organized with an introduction and rationale for electronically controlled delivery technology. The underlying principles are then described. The applications of these principles to commercial and novel technologies are elucidated.

1.2 FUNDAMENTALS OF THE TECHNOLOGIES

The time of administration of certain drugs has been demonstrated to be critical to either safety or efficacy. As elaborated in Chapter 2 by Hrushesky, this is particularly true of cancer chemotherapy. The devastating side effects of chemotherapy may be substantially mitigated by administering the drugs in late evening. Given the traditional 9-to-5 hours for clinical practice, therapeutic application has not reflected this discovery. Perhaps appropriately designed drug delivery systems or adroit use of melatonin or light therapy to shift patients' circadian rhythms is in order.

Internal physiological factors may also modulate the pharmacological response. Tolerance and on–off fluctuations have been demonstrated to occur in all dopaminergic-based therapies.[3] Optimization of chronotherapy has not been systematically studied. Continuous administration of transdermal nitroglycerin led to tolerance, and, consequently, patients remove the patch at night to maintain efficacy.[4] Ronald Burnette in Chapter 5 has attempted a general pharmacokinetic–pharmacodynamic model of temporal delivery. By using a temporally modulated drug input in an EC50 model with interindividual variation, the maximization of efficacy can be interpreted in terms of adjusting the phase shifts between the drug input and the circadian rhythm.

The barrier properties of the stratum corneum are the initial motivation for the technologies of iontophoresis, sonophoresis, and electroporation. Understanding of the ohmic properties of skin at low current densities and the nonlinear effects due to electro-osmosis at practical current densities can be important for optimizing these systems. The electrical properties of skin are reviewed in Chapter 3 by Jagdish Singh et al., and the implications for iontophoresis are discussed. As discussed by Amin and Maibach in Chapter 4, skin tolerability may be a limiting factor for all skin-related noninvasive technologies. Irritation testing in rabbits and guinea pig sensitization are the basic toxicological methods for evaluating these effects. This must be followed by analogous studies in humans. The work of Molitor[5] indicates that skin irritation from iontophoresis is related to pH changes resulting from the use of platinum electrodes exposed to greater than 1 V. More recent data are, however, quite promising, and appropriately designed electrodes exhibit minimal erythema at practical current densities for several-hour exposures.[6]

A review by Sietse Wouters in Chapter 6 of miniaturized electronics and true microelectronics for drug delivery systems shows both the potential state of the art and the limitations of the current applications. For convenience and cost, conventional battery technologies and miniaturization have been employed in first-generation systems. Microelectronics and micromachining are in the prototype stage for certain infusion pumps and in academic studies of "intelligent" oral drug delivery systems.

1.3 APPLICATIONS

Infusion pumps have reached commercial reality at the home use level. Such pumps are typically used to obtain levels of therapeutic control in extreme cases that could not be achieved by other means. In particular, pumps are used routinely in diabetics and with baclofen to achieve around-the-clock control over spasticity. These pumps are still bulky and are accepted by a limited, motivated patient population. With large markets, the costs of microelectronics and micromachining plummet, and more user-friendly devices are being achieved. In some applications, the volume of the drug reservoir becomes the limiting factor in terms of size. Numerous applications of infusion pumps to the CNS area have been documented in the literature,[7] and these are leading to several specialized niche therapies. Kenneth Heruth in Chapter 9 has reviewed the application of the SynchroMed infusion pump to baclofen for spasticity and discussed its future potential use in patients with Alzheimer's disease.

Iontophoresis is the most advanced of the "noninvasive" electronically controlled drug delivery technologies. In addition to the previously mentioned Phase III trials, bioavailability trials of a few peptides have been published.[8,9] The lack of oral bioavailability and the short half-life of peptides and proteins make them ideal candidates for novel drug delivery, in particular, iontophoresis, sonophoresis or phonophoresis, and electroporation. Estimates of the radii of pores for ion transport through skin from thermodynamic models[10] range from 20 to 30 Å, and, therefore, skin presents a likely route for peptide delivery. However, the potentially antigenic properties of peptides and proteins may result in many cases of sensitization, because the skin has the most exquisitely sensitive immune system in the body. Delgado-Charro and Guy in Chapter 7 have provided an extensive review of the literature of iontophoretic peptide delivery, which appears to be one of the most promising applications.

Many physiological factors can create the need for complex chronotherapy. In addition to circadian rhythms, diseases such as diabetic control of glucose are complicated by external factors, for example, diet and exercise, that can create profound variations in the level of blood glucose. In the DCCT trial,[11] it was shown that monitoring the level of glucose at least seven times daily and adjusting the dose of insulin significantly reduced the incidence of the deleterious complications of diabetes. However, from such tight control of blood glucose, the number of hypoglycemic incidents can increase. Noninvasive monitoring of glucose by iontophoresis, as discussed by Janet Tamada and Russell Potts, in Chapter 8, can overcome both of these difficulties. Clinical trials in patients with diabetes with a practical electrochemical biosensor in a wristwatch have begun.

1.4   NOVEL TECHNOLOGIES

Sonophoresis and electroporation are noninvasive technologies in their developmental infancy. While sonophoresis, or phonophoresis, the use of ultrasound to enhance drug delivery, has been discussed in the literature for many years, the enhancements observed were subtle compared with iontophoresis and did not justify the investment in developing that technology beyond iontophoresis. Joseph Kost reviews sonophoretic drug delivery in Chapter 11. More recently, lower frequencies have been investigated, and much more sizable enhancements have been observed. The mechanism is not clear, but could involve either phase transitions or even resonance with the structures in skin. This has kindled interest in peptide delivery and glucose monitoring by sonophoresis. The practicalities of *in vivo* delivery have not yet been investigated, and skin tolerability under repetitive applications needs to be defined. However, the early data are quite intriguing.

Electroporation or the creation of pores through skin at high voltages is the most novel skin-related technology, and its application to gene therapy is being investigated. Mark Prausnitz in Chapter 10 presents some astonishing increases in skin transport *in vitro*. While the literature has some scattered work on *in vivo* effects, systematic studies of pain and skin tolerability from electroporation have not been performed. Commercial application of this technology is probably the most remote.

1.5   CONCLUSION

Strides toward commercialization of infusion pumps and iontophoretic systems for home use therapy are providing therapeutic advantages in everyday life that were previously limited to a few patients in hospital settings. Given the combined requirements for clinical evaluation of the device and the drug for home use, the progress has been remarkable. At the same time, innovation in medicine and technology needs to continue with ever increasing speed to improve the quality of life.

REFERENCES

1. W.J.M. Hrushesky, The multifrequency (circadian fertility cycle, and season) balance between host and cancer, In W.J.M. Hrushesky, R. Langer, and F. Theeuwes, Eds., *Temporal Control of Drug Delivery, Ann. N.Y. Acad. Sci.,* 618:228–256 (1991).
2. R. von Roemling, The therapeutic index of cytotoxic chemotherapy depends upon circadian drug timing. In W.J.M. Hrushesky, R. Langer, and F. Theeuwes, Eds., *Temporal Control of Drug Delivery, Ann. N.Y. Acad. Sci.,* 618:292–311 (1991).
3. S.M.Stahl, Applications of new drug delivery technologies to Parkinson's disease and dopaminergic agents. *J. Neural Transm. Suppl.* 27:123–132 (1988).
4. S. Scardi, F. Camerini, C. Pandullo, G. Pollavini, and the Collaborative Nitro Group, Efficacy of continuous and intermittent transdermal treatment with nitroglycerin in effort angina pectoris: a multicentric study. *Int. J. Cardiol.* 32:241–248 (1991).
5. H. Molitor, Pharmacological aspects of drug administration by ion-transfer. The Merck Report 22-29 (1943).
6. R.van der Geest, D.A.R. Elshove, M. Danhof, A.P.M. Lavrijsen, and H.E. Bodde, Non-invasive assessment of skin barrier integrity and skin irritation following ionto-phoretic current application in humans. *J. Controlled Release* 41:205–213 (1996).
7. S. Kroin, R.D. Penn, R. C. Beissinger, and R.C. Arzbaecher, *Exp. Brain Res.* 54:191 (1984).
8. J.D. DeNuzzio, R. Bock, A. McFarland, M. O'Connell, P. Palaer, and B. Sage. *In vivo* iontophoretic delivery and pharmacokinetics of peptides. *Proc. Int. Symp. Control. Rel. Bioact. Mater.* 22:684–685 (1995).
9. K. Boericke, M.A. O'Connell, R. Bock, P. Green, and J.A. Down, Iontophoretic delivery of human parathyroiud hormone (1-34) in swine, *Proc. Int. Symp. Control. Rel. Bioact. Mater.* 23:200–201 (1996).
10. S.M.Dinh, C. W. Luo, and B. Berner, Upper and lower limits of human skin electrical resistance in iontophoresis, *AIChE J.* 39:2011–2018 (1993).
11. The Diabetes Control and Complications Trial Research Group, The effect of intensive treatment of diabetes on the development of long-term complications in insulin-dependent diabetes mellitus. *N. Engl. J. Med.* 329:977 (1993).

2 Home-Based Circadian-Optimized Cancer Chemotherapy

William J. M. Hrushesky

CONTENTS

This work was supported, in part, by NIH R01 CA 31635 "Clinical Applications of Chronobiology to Cancer Medicine" and by VA Merit Review awards to William J. M. Hrushesky. This chapter contains both original material and sections of prior published materials, all of which have been authored by Dr. Hrushesky, who is a full-time U.S. government employee. Thereby, this work is not and cannot be copyrighted.

Abstract — Traditionally, drug delivery has meant getting a simple chemical absorbed predictably from the gut or from the site of injection. A second-generation drug delivery goal has been the perfection of continuous constant rate (zero-order) delivery of simple xenobiotic molecules or common hormones. Living organisms are not "zero-order" in their requirement for or response to drugs. They are predictably resonating dynamic systems which require different amounts of drug at different times in order to maximize desired and minimize undesired drug effects.

Soon, many "drugs" will not be simple, but complex, delicate, extremely powerful protein molecules which must be delivered within a narrow concentration range to a specific site at an optimal time or in an optimal temporal infusion pattern.

Clinical trials testing circadian specified treatment of 120 patients with cancer with the two-drug combination of doxorubicin/cisplatin required more than 1000 hospital admissions and more than 3000 hospital days. These studies demonstrate the fact that anticancer drug toxicity and resultant dose intensity, tumor control, and patient survival are each dependent upon treatment timing. Subsequently, 300 patients with cancer have received precisely timed circadian-modified continuous 5-fluoro-2'-deoxyuridine (FUDR) infusion for up to 3 years using an implanted computerized delivery system. This chronotherapy was delivered on an entirely outpatient basis and with extreme precision. These outpatient studies further corroborate the circadian dependence of drug toxicity and dose intensity. The further practical application of chronobiology to cancer medicine absolutely requires the further development of intelligent open- and closed-loop delivery systems.

2.1 INTRODUCTION

In 1972, a paper appeared in *Science* which reported that the arrangement within the day of three-hourly doses of cytosine arabinoside (Ara-C) had a pronounced effect on the survival rate of mice inoculated with L1210 leukemia cells.[1] This study was built on extensive prior work demonstrating that all Ara-C toxicities are markedly dependent on the time, in the day/night cycle, at which the drug is administered.[2] Together, the experiments showed unequivocally that, in mice, the timing of Ara-C administration predictably modulates its therapeutic index.

Surprisingly, nearly 20 years later, this simple hypothesis has still not been extended to clinical trials for human leukemia, even though the mainstay treatment for the most common deadly acute leukemia has remained Ara-C, used at higher and higher dose intensity with greater and greater toxicity.[3] In the meantime, it has been shown that all anthracyclines, which are generally coupled with Ara-C to treat the nonlymphocytic leukemias, also exhibit a pronounced circadian time dependency in their pharmacology, toxicology, and efficacy in mice and in humans.[4-6] Furthermore, many combination chemotherapy studies, done in follow-up to the initial Ara-C study, have demonstrated that the addition of a second or third drug to the regimen seldom interferes with the enhancement in therapeutic index resulting from circadian optimization of each drug.[7]

A personal background of clinical experience with high-dose cytoxan in G. W. Santos' pioneering bone marrow transplant unit and with ultrahigh-dose-intensity chemotherapy for small-cell lung cancer as a member of the National Cancer Institute (NCI) solid tumor service made it impossible for me to ignore the likely clinical import of diminishing the toxicity and increasing the efficacy of the drugs available to us by any means, including optimal circadian timing. In Minnesota, we began a series of studies in rodents that led to the circadian optimization of the doxorubicin/cisplatin combination.[8] NCI-sponsored randomized clinical studies then revealed that each and every doxorubicin and cisplatin toxicity is largely dependent upon the circadian timing of these agents in human beings.[4,9] In patients with widespread ovarian cancer, optimal circadian drug timing resulted in safer administration of higher doses of drug and, in turn, a fourfold improvement in the 5-year survival rate of women with advanced ovarian cancer.[10] These clinical studies have also remained largely ignored.

In the early 1980s, work in mice defined the fact that 5-fluorouracil (5-FU) toxicology is circadian stage dependent.[11] The LD_{50} of this commonly used mainstay of solid tumor treatment is markedly and reproducibly higher when given in the sleep span.[12] Peters et al.[13] confirmed this early work and extended it to show that nonlethal 5-FU toxicity and tumor control of a murine colon cancer are each dependent upon circadian 5-FU timing.

Chronotoxicology studies of intravenous and intraperitoneal bolus FUDR administration in mice revealed that the safest time for this drug was several hours earlier in the day than for fluorouracil.[14] The highest LD_{50} (lowest toxicity) occurred reproducibly late in the daily activity span. The half-life of FUDR is extremely short; it must therefore be used clinically by protracted infusion. This fact made us reluctant to undertake clinical studies based solely upon bolus studies in the mouse. In order to allow better prediction of optimal circadian FUDR infusion shape, continuous infusion studies were performed upon Fisher 344 rats bearing the fluoropyrimidine-sensitive 13762 adenocarcinoma. These studies revealed that continuous FUDR infusions weighted with peak delivery rates at different circadian times are reproducibly more or less toxic and more or less effective than continuous flat FUDR infusions.[15] It was found that continuous FUDR infusions weighted toward the end of daily activity and the first half of the daily sleep span are reproducibly less toxic and more effective than flat infusions or infusions of the same shape but peaking at other times during the day.[15]

2.2 DETERMINATION OF THE THERAPEUTIC INDEX OF FLOXURIDINE BY ITS CIRCADIAN INFUSION PATTERN

To test if circadian timing of a drug is important for its toxicity and antitumor activity, we compared the circadian patterns observed with seven equal doses of floxuridine (FUDR) infused either at a variable rate or at a constant rate in female F344 rats. For the variable rate infusion, the daily dose of FUDR was divided into four 6-h portions of 68, 15, 2, and 15% to achieve a quasi-sinusoidal pattern. Peak drug delivery occurred during one of six different times of day. At a dose level resulting in 50% overall mortality, lethal toxicity differed significantly, depending upon the circadian stage of maximum drug delivery.

Depending on the circadian stage of maximum drug flow, variable rate infusions were more toxic than or as toxic as constant rate infusion. FUDR lethality was lowest when constant rate infusion was used or when variable rate infusion peaked during the late activity--early rest span of the recipients (Figure 2.1). The circadian pattern of variable-rate infusion also determined the antitumor activity in tumor-bearing rats. At a therapeutic dose level and at identical dose intensity, the variable rate infusion pattern, with peak drug flow during the late activity–early rest span, resulted in significantly greater delay and the only demonstrated actual tumor shrinkage in tumor growth observed with either the constant rate infusion or other variable rate patterns (Figure 2.2). We conclude that the toxicity and antitumor activity of FUDR depend on the circadian timing of the infusion peak when the drug is given by variable rate infusion. Since some of the circadian-shaped infusions studied are toxicologically and therapeutically inferior to constant rate infusion, the circadian pattern and not the quasi intermittency of circadian FUDR administration is primarily responsible for these pharmacodynamic differences.[15]

As a practical matter, in aggregate, these data suggest that the optimal shape of FUDR infusion should peak 4 to 6 h later than was originally extrapolated from bolus studies. If the day is divided into quadrants, these data suggest that the optimal peak infusion time is most likely to be between 9 p.m. and 3 a.m. All clinical comparisons have shown infusions peaking 4 to 6 h earlier than this to be substantially less toxic than constant rate infusion. These data indicate that even more benefit

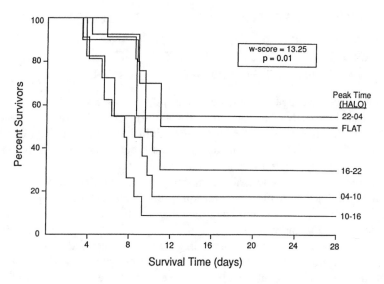

FIGURE 2.1   Life table analysis for FUDR continuous infusion.

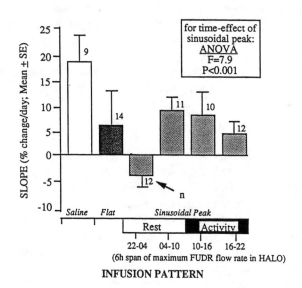

FIGURE 2.2   Flat vs. sinusoidal FUDR Infusion. Day 6 tumor response (slope) in female Fischer rats following 48 h of equal dose (700 mg/kg).

might accrue if the daily infusion peak was delayed 4 to 6 h. This possibility urgently awaits additional clinical study. Unfortunately, these data were unavailable prior to the design and execution of the Phase I clinical study reported in the November 1989, *Journal of Clinical Oncology* and outlined below.[16]

2.3   CIRCADIAN PATTERNING OF CONTINUOUS FLOXURIDINE INFUSION REDUCES TOXICITY AND ALLOWS HIGHER DOSE INTENSITY IN PATIENTS WITH WIDESPREAD CANCER

Continuous long-term FUDR infusion frequently causes severe and dose-limiting gastrointestinal toxicity when administered at a constant rate at commonly prescribed dose levels. In preclinical studies, a circadian infusion pattern peaking late in the daily activity phase was better tolerated and had superior antitumor activity than a constant infusion against a transplanted tumor. Based upon these data and upon other chronobiological cytokinetic and pharmacological considerations, we compared a circadian patterned variable rate infusion with a maximal flow rate in the late afternoon/early evening and minimum flow rate during the early morning hours to a constant rate infusion in 54 patients with widespread cancer. All FUDR infusions were administered using an implanted drug pump (Synchromed,® Medtronic Corporation). In a pilot crossover study and a second randomized trial, patients with metastatic malignancies treated with equal dose intensities experienced less frequent and less severe diarrhea, nausea, and vomiting following variable-rate infusion. In a third study, the dose intensity of variable rate infusion was escalated stepwise to determine the maximum-tolerated dose. Patients receiving time-modified FUDR infusion tolerated an average of 1.45-fold more drug per unit time while evincing minimal toxicity. FUDR infusion was found to have activity against progressive metastatic renal cell cancer (RCC). Increased dose intensity achieved by optimal circadian shaping may improve the therapeutic index of infusional FUDR and may help control malignancies that are refractory to conventional chemotherapy.

2.4   CROSSOVER STUDY

The purpose of this initial crossover study was to determine if patients with severe toxicity after constant rate infusion could tolerate the same dose level after changing the infusion pattern from constant to variable rate. All patients were started on flat rate infusion using Synchromed pumps and received an average of 2.2 treatment courses (range, one to three) at a mean dose intensity of (mean ± SE) 0.45 ± 0.08 mg/kg/week. This form of therapy had to be stopped due to the appearance of severe toxicity in five of six patients. After full recovery from toxicity, which lasted 6 weeks in one case, each patient was crossed over to treatment with a variable rate infusion. They each subsequently received an average of 4.5 additional courses with variable rate infusion at a slightly higher mean dose intensity of 0.46 ± 0.1 mg/kg/week ($t = 0.32$; $P = 0.75$ from comparison of flat vs. variable rate dose intensity). Only two of six patients had mild diarrhea, while moderate to severe diarrhea, which had occurred in five of six patients during flat infusion, did not occur at all on variable rate infusion (Table 2.1). Nausea and vomiting were less frequent and less severe than with constant rate infusion. Analysis of the frequency of nausea and vomiting per courses given revealed 54 vs. 18% for constant and variable rate infusion, respectively ($X^2 = 4.0$; $P < 0.05$). These data demonstrate that individuals

TABLE 2.1
Circadian Fluoropyrimidine Infusion
Equal Dosing: Gastrointestinal Toxicity as Function of Infusion Pattern

	Infusion Rate		
	Constant	Variable	X^2
Number of patients	14	16	
Number of courses	29	57	
Nausea/vomiting			
Grade 1	50%	19%	$0.05 < P < 0.10$
Grade 2	0%	0%	
Diarrhea[a]			
Grade 1	43%	6%	$P < 0.02$
Grade 2	36%	0%	$P < 0.01$
Grade 3	14%	0%	$P < 0.1$
Toxicity-related hopsital admissions	21%	0%	$0.05 < P < 0.1$

[a] Incidence per patient group.

tolerate the same dose intensity of FUDR when given as a variable rate circadian time-specified infusion with significantly less severe and less frequent gastrointestinal toxicity when a constant rate infusion is employed.

2.5 RANDOMIZED TOXICITY COMPARISON

In the study, 30 patients were randomized between constant rate (29 evaluable treatment courses) and variable rate FUDR infusion (57 evaluable courses). The starting FUDR dose level of 0.15 mg/kg/day was maintained if permitted by toxicity (no dose escalation), and the treatment continued until tumor progression. Patients on constant rate infusion received an average of 2.2 ± 0.4 treatment courses; those on variable rate infusion received 3.6 ± 0.8 courses. Dose intensity was equal for both groups (0.446 ± 0.1 vs. 0.483 ± 0.1 mg/kg/week of FUDR for constant rate and variable rate, respectively; $t = 1.7$; $P = 0.10$). There was, however, a large difference in the severity and frequency of toxicity (Table 2.2). Fifty percent of patients on constant rate infusion had nausea and vomiting vs. 19% on time-modified infusion. Ninety-three percent of those on constant rate infusion had diarrhea of mild to severe grade vs. 6% of the patients on variable rate, whose toxicity was only mild. Hospitalizations were required only for intravenous rehydration in 21% of the patients after constant rate infusion. Regardless of schedule of treatment, the onset of toxicity started during the second week of the treatment. In some cases, the onset occurred later in the first half of the 14-day, treatment-free interval. Early vs. delayed onset did not correlate with severity of toxicity. In most patients, the duration of toxicity was brief (<3 days) and mild toxicity was occasionally not recognized as treatment related by the patients, but rather interpreted as "flu."

TABLE 2.2
Dose Escalation: Gastrointestinal Toxicity

	Dose (mg/kg/day)			
	0.15	0.175	0.20	0.225 to 0.35
Number of patients	38	24	19	10
Nausea/vomiting[a]				
Grade 1	29%	29%	16%	10%
Grade 2	0%	4%	5%	0%
Diarrhea[a]				
Grade 1	16%	13%	0%	0%
Grade 2	3%	4%	5%	0%
Grade 3	3%	0%	0%	0%
Toxicity-related hospital admissions[a]	6%	0%	5%	0%

[a] Incidence per patient group.

In both groups, bone marrow toxicity was not observed. Peripheral blood counts, which were determined every 2 weeks, remained within normal ranges. Similarly, liver function tests (SGOT, alkaline phosphatase, and lactic dehydrogenase), kidney function tests, and serum electrolytes did not change in the absence of tumor progression. No acute or cumulative cardiac toxicity was observed. The treatment did not result in alopecia, skin alterations, or the "hand-foot" syndrome frequently associated with prolonged fluorouracil infusion nor was there any evidence for neurotoxicity. Data from this study suggest that the dose-limiting toxicities of 0.15 mg/kg/day of FUDR can be greatly reduced by time modification of the infusion pattern.

2.6 DOSE ESCALATION STUDY

In this study, 39 patients were accrued to this infusion pattern. The starting dose of 0.15 mg/kg/day was escalated each month by 0.25 mg/kg/day if permitted by toxicity. Of the 39 patients 1 was not evaluable for toxicity because of concurrent radiation therapy to his abdomen. Of the remaining patients, 71% did not have toxicity and qualified for dose escalation. However, only 63% were escalated. The remaining 8% of patients had rapid tumor progression and were taken off study. Of that 63%, 50% reached the second escalation step, and 26% were available for further escalation. The highest dose achieved through this stepwise escalation was 0.325 mg/kg/day × 14 days. Mean dose intensity was 0.645 ± 0.1 mg/kg/week of FUDR for the entire group. This compares to 0.446 ± 0.1 vs. 0.483 ± .1 mg/kg/week of FUDR for constant rate and variable rate infusion, respectively, in patients who participated in the above randomized study and who did not have dose escalations. It represents a 45% increase in mean dose intensity over the maximum-tolerated constant rate infusion level. Secondary to the patient selection with dose escalation, the incidence of toxicity remained low (less than one third of the patients had side effects after each of the escalation steps) and the toxicity grades remained low. Even at high dose intensity, cumulative drug toxicity was absent for bone marrow, heart, kidney, lungs, and liver. Although 11 patients received treatment for more than a year, neurological alterations or skin changes were not observed. These data indicate that higher-dose-intensity continuous infusion can be safely given if the infusion is patterned so that most of the daily dose is given late in the day.[16]

2.7 CIRCADIAN-SHAPED INFUSIONS OF FUDR FOR PROGRESSIVE METASTATIC RENAL CELL CARCINOMA (RCC)

Between March 1985 and November 1988, 68 unselected patients with progressive metastatic RCC were treated with continuous infusion FUDR. Of these patients, 37% had previously received and failed systemic treatment. By using implantable pumps for automatic drug delivery, FUDR was continuously infused for 14 days at monthly intervals. Starting dose was 0.15 mg/kg/day (intravenous; $n = 61$) or 0.25 mg/kg/day (intra-arterial; $n = 7$); intravenous doses were increased or decreased in increments of 0.025 mg/kg/day as permitted by toxicity. Diarrhea (with or without mild abdominal cramping) and nausea/vomiting limited the FUDR intravenous infusion, and hepatic function abnormalities limited FUDR intra-arterial infusion. The use of a circadian-modified infusion schedule permitted high FUDR doses to be safely given as compared with a constant rate infusion schedule. Of 63 patients evaluable for response, 56 received systemic FUDR infusion. As depicted in Figure 2.3, their median survival on treatment was 14 months. Four durable complete responses with a median duration of 33 months (CR = 7.1%), and seven partial responses with a median duration of 25 months (PR = 12.5%) were observed — objective response rate CR + PR = $19.6 \pm 5.1\%$ (95% confidence limits). Four additional patients had minor tumor responses (MR = 7.1%). The survival probability of each major response group is shown in Figure 2.3. In a subgroup of seven evaluable patients receiving hepatic arterial FUDR for rapidly progressive RCC metastatic to the liver, we observed one complete and three partial responses (CR + PR = $57.2 \pm 42.8\%$). The median survival of this particularly bad prognostic group was 16 months. Overall, objective response (CR + PR) was seen in a quarter of evaluable patients treated: 15 of 63.

While only 15 of the 63 evaluable patients (25.4%) have had objective tumor progression, the median follow-up time for all 68 patients was 28 months (range 1 to 42), and their median survival duration is 15 months (range of 3 to 37 months) (Figure 2.4). It is concluded from these data that continuous chronobiologically modified infusion FUDR is an effective outpatient treatment for progressive metastatic RCC producing durable tumor response and causing little toxicity. Subsequent infusional FUDR data in the rat model would predict better results when the infusion is peaked 4 to 6 h later each day.[17]

In summary, patients receiving time-modified FUDR infusion tolerated an average of 1.45-fold more drug per unit time while evincing minimal toxicity. FUDR

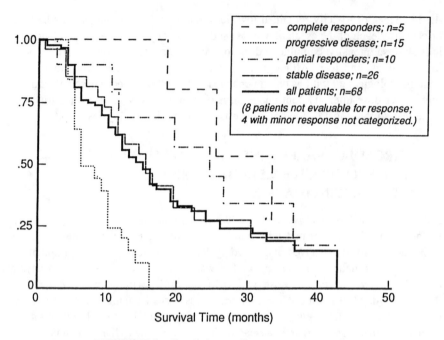

FIGURE 2.3   Survival according to response status.

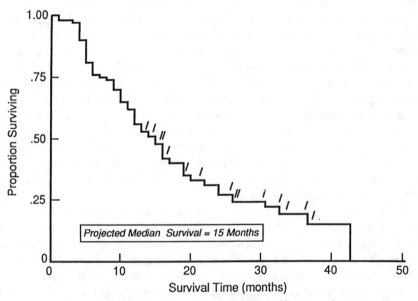

Survival duration of all 68 consecutive patients with progressive metastatic
renal cell carcinoma receiving continuous FUDR infusion therapy.

FIGURE 2.4   Survival duration of all 68 consecutive patients with progressive metastatic
RCC receiving continuous FUDR infusion therapy.

infusion was found to have activity against progressive metastatic RCC. We concluded that increased dose intensity achieved by "optimal" circadian shaping may improve the therapeutic index of infusional FUDR and may help control malignancies that are refractory to conventional chemotherapy. Given the subsequent preclinical information, a suboptimally designed randomized Phase I–II clinical study investigating whether intrahepatic FUDR toxicities are lessened and whether dose intensity can be safely increased by "optimally" shaping the FUDR infusion in circadian time has also produced positive results in 50 of the cancer patients randomized to circadian or flat infusion.[18] So far, clinical advantage has been demonstrated for "optimal" circadian drug timing for systemic FUDR infusion in patients with metastatic RCC;[17] for intrahepatic infusion of FUDR for the treatment of colorectal cancer metastatic to liver;[19] and Leví et al.[20] have demonstrated advantage to shaping 5-FU infusion (to peak at 4 a.m.) in patients with widespread colorectal cancer. Our present murine results lead us, however, to conclude that we may not have tested the "optimal" circadian shape. Were the clinical Phase I comparisons to be initiated today, a peak infusion span 4 to 6 h later in the day than the peak time chosen for the original clinical studies (between 8 or 9 p.m. and 2 or 3 a.m., not between 3 p.m. and 9 p.m.) would be selected. This possible missing of the best treatment timing illustrates the risk of two-armed study designs extrapolated from murine experiments.

2.8 CHRONOPHARMACOLOGY AND CIRCADIAN TIME–DEPENDENT BIOCHEMICAL PHARMACOLOGY

Attempts to define the mechanisms by which the pharmacodynamics of 5-FU or fluorodeoxyuridine vary reproducibly with circadian times have begun. Mechanisms of potential importance to the circadian time dependency of fluoropyrimidine toxicity and anticancer activity may relate (1) to the way drugs are handled by the organs primarily responsible for catabolism or excretion (drug pharmacology); (2) to the way the drugs are handled by the cellular targets of toxicity (biochemical pharmacology); or (3) to correlatively the cell cycle phase that target cells are likely to be inhabiting at different times of day when a cell cycle stage specific drug exposure occurs (circadian cytokinetics). Several recent publications have investigated the biochemical mechanisms of circadian stage dependency of fluoropyrimidine toxicology.

The pharmacology of continuous constant rate 5-FU infusion, as reflected by rhythmically varying drug levels over the day, was first demonstrated by Petit et al.[21] and later by Harris et al.[22] Each group noted markedly different pharmacokinetics at different times of day. The fact that the timing of peak FU levels differed in the two groups of patients may relate to the fact that the French patients received cisplatin at a fixed time of day prior to each 5-day 5-FU infusion while the American patients received 5-FU only and for much longer spans. This peak difference opens the question of circadian stage dependent cisplatin/5-FU interaction which deserves further preclinical and clinical study. The major points of each paper, however, remain the clear observation of large, within-study, and cross-subject reproducible differences in drug level at different times of days during a continuous constant rate 5-FU infusion.

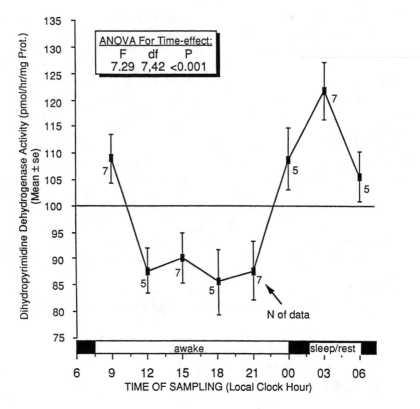

FIGURE 2.5 Circadian waveform of DRD activity in blood mononuclear cells of seven healthy subjects (four women; three men). (Data expressed as percent of mean.)

Tuchman et al.[23] and then Diasio et al.[24] demonstrated the importance of dihydropyrimidine dehydrogenase (DPD) as the rate-limiting catabolic enzyme in the breakdown of 5-FU to nontoxic metabolites. Furthermore, on a tissue level, when human peripheral blood mononuclear cells were isolated around the clock in seven subjects, we found that DPD levels were much higher just after usual sleep onset than at other times of the day (see Figure 2.5 and Table 2.3).[25] In their recent elegant *ex vivo* rat liver perfusion study, Harris et al.[26] demonstrate unequivocally that 5-FU clearance and metabolism by the liver are critically circadian stage dependent. Eight times as much 5-FU was extracted per unit time by the isolated perfused rat liver tested in mid to late sleep compared with livers removed and perfused in mid activity.[26] Our DPD data showing mononuclear DPD peaking in sleep are very consistent with these murine extraction data and with murine hepatic DPD activity circadian pattern.[25] In aggregate, these data suggest that a prominent circadian rhythm in DPD activity of both organs or metabolism as well as cells more peripheral to 5-FU catabolism may be responsible, at least in some part, for the circadian dependence of 5-FU toxicity in rat, mouse, and human being and perhaps also for the circadian dependence of its anticancer efficacy documented in rat and mouse models and more lately suggested by work in humans.

TABLE 2.3
Subject and Data Characteristics and Results of Cosinor Analyses

Subject	Sex	Age	N Data	Range (low, high) (pmol/h/mg prot)	ROC[a] (%)	Results from Fit of 24-h Cosine (Single Cosinor)			
						P	MESOR ± SE (pmol/h/mg prot)	Amp ± SE	Acrophase ± SE (h & min)[b]
RL	F	41	8	6113, 12155	98.8	0.002	8640 ± 253	2765 ± 358	00:34 ± 00:28
CH	F	25	8	6792, 11416	68.1	0.082	9441 ± 363	1505 ± 514	02:11 ± 01:20
DM	F	26	8	5744, 9814	70.9	0.319	7674 ± 435	1048 ± 615	01:16 ± 02:16
KJ	F	19	4	4871, 9164	88.1	0.043	7933 ± 075	3032 ± 135	01:42 ± 00:08
RS	M	40	4	4779, 6600	38.1	0.446	5757 ± 326	1063 ± 565	23:13 ± 01:28
JN	M	27	8	8122, 14154	74.3	0.083	10914 ± 489	2019 ± 691	01:44 ± 01:20
JR	M	24	8	9352, 14776	58.0	0.379	10916 ± 594	1294 ± 840	22:02 ± 02:28

Group Rhythm Summary by Population Mean Cosinor

No. of Subjects	P	Amplitude (95% limits)	Acrophase (95% limits)
7 using original units	0.007	1723 (590, 2960)	00:56 (21:52, 02:24)
7 using Amp as % MESOR	0.009	20.2 (6.3, 35.1)	00:56 (21:48, 02:24)

a ROC = range of change from lowest to highest value.
b Acrophase referenced to local midnight.

The circadian pharmacology and cellular biochemical pharmacology of fluoro-deoxyuridine is less clearly established than that of 5-FU, in part, because it is administered in much lower milligram amounts, requiring much more sensitive analytical methods. This picture is also complicated by the fact that these two fluoropyrimidines are interconvertible. Roemeling et al.[27] has preliminarily observed a twofold circadian difference in the convertibility of FUDR to 5-FU, indicating that FUDR pharmacodynamics may depend upon the circadian DPD rhythms at some times of the day but not at others. The activities of other enzymes of prominent importance in the activation of FUDR to fluorouracil dehydromonophosphate (FdUMP), dihydrouracil dehydrogenase, uridine phosphorylase, and thymidine phosphorylase have each been shown to be circadian rhythmic in mouse liver;[28] however, the exact contribution of the circadian time structure of the activities of these enzymes to the crisp, high-amplitude circadian rhythm in FUDR toxicity and efficacy requires further work in murine and human systems. No information is currently available about the circadian pattern of thymidylate synthase (TS) activity, which is the primary enzymatic target of FdUMP in either tumor or host tissues.

All in all, these preclinical and clinical fluoropyrimidine results indicate that circadian time structure in the organs of catabolism and excretion and the biochemical enzyme activity rhythms in normal or malignant target cells may each be critically important in determining the optimal time of day for bolus drug adminis-tration or the optimal circadian shape of continuous infusion fluoropyrimidine ther-apy. As the metabolic processes necessary to catabolize these two drugs are different yet related and the intracellular targets are overlapping but to some extent distinct, the two agents have distinct optimal circadian timings that are nearly a third of a day apart.[14]

2.9   CIRCADIAN CELL CYCLE GATING

In addition to the circadian pattern of activity of important cellular biochemical pathways, circadian patterns of cytokinetic activity in malignant and nonmalignant tissues damaged by these drugs may be of equal importance in explaining the circadian pharmacodynamics. Both of these agents are most active against dividing cells during the process of DNA synthesis. DNA synthesis in all tissues studied throughout the circadian cycle is nonrandomly distributed throughout the day.[29] Depending upon dose and duration of infusion, the gut, skin, and/or bone marrow are the primary targets of fluoropyrimidine toxicity. Human skin,[30] bone marrow,[31,32] and human colorectal mucosa have each been demonstrated to be markedly circadian rhythmic in the amount of ongoing DNA synthesis.[33] When FUDR is infused with the lower rate during early morning hours, the clinical toxicity is markedly dimin-ished and dose intensity can be safely elevated. In the human being, the dose-limiting target of FUDR infusional toxicity is the colorectal mucosa. In our recent work, serial biopsies, every 3 h, of rectal mucosa for 24 h from 24 human volunteers in both the fed and fasted states reveal that there is much greater *in vitro* tritiated thymidine uptake occurring in colonic epithelial cells removed during the early morning hours (4 h prior to usual awakening) than later in the day and evening (see Figure 2.6).[34] This circadian stage coincidence of the time of day of lowest tritiated

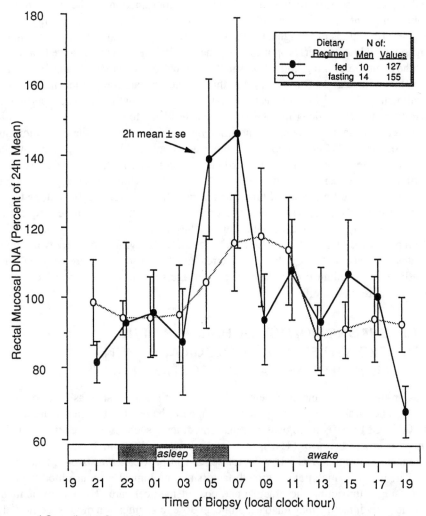

FIGURE 2.6   Circadian waveform of rectal mucosal cell DNA synthesis in 16 clinically healthy men on fed or fasting regimen. Sampling at 2- or 3-h intervals for 24 h beginning at either 0900 or 2100 (2-hourly means for each group obtained after first reexpressing individual data series as percent of mean.)

thymidine epithelial cell uptake and daily time of lowest FUDR colonic epithelial toxicity is intriguing.

Few data are available to evaluate whether or not spontaneous human malignancies are cytokinetically coordinated on the circadian timescale. The most thorough evaluation of this difficult question has been accomplished in patients with ovarian cancer. Klevecz et al.[35] sampled cells washed from the peritoneal cavities of a large number of women, every 2 to 4 h, for up to 4 days. Using sophisticated cytofluorometric techniques, these investigators found circadian coordination of the proportion of both malignant epithelial and nonmalignant mesothelial cells synthesizing DNA. Higher proportions of malignant cells were actively synthesizing DNA in the morning hours while higher proportions of mesothelial cells were engaged in DNA synthesis in the evening hours.[35] A smaller number of patients with non-Hodgkin's lymphoma have undergone, every 4 h, thin needle aspiration of tumor masses for a minimum of 24 h. While no clear population circadian rhythm in the proportion of cytofluorometrically determined S-phase cells has been found, some individuals do, however, have large time-dependent differences which cluster in the early morning hours of the day.[36] Serial biopsies of tumor and normal skin in one of our patients with widespread cutaneous epidermoid carcinoma reveal high-amplitude circadian rhythms in mitotic index of her tumor cell population with the same phase as her normal skin. Mitotic indices of tumor and normal tissues were identical at the times of daily lowest values, while tumor cell mitoses were manyfold more frequent at times in the day associated with the usual highest daily mitotic activity (manuscript in preparation). All of these limited data suggest that the cytokinetic activity of tumor tissues is likely to be coordinated in circadian time and that there may well be windows in circadian time when cell cycle stage specific attacks upon these cells may be more or less effective.

2.10   CHRONOBIOLOGY OF HEMATOPOIETIC GROWTH FACTORS, BIOLOGICAL RESPONSE MODIFIERS, AND ADRENOCORTICOTROPINS

This group of agents includes hematopoietic growth factors, such as erythropoietin (EPO) and granulocyte and granulocyte/macrophage colony-stimulating factor (G-CSF, GM-CSF), biological response modifiers, such as interleukin-2 (IL-2), tumor necrosis factor-α (TNF), and interferons, and protein hormones, such as adrenocorticotropins (ACTH), somatotropins, and peptide agonists or antagonists.

The use of hematopoietic growth factors and biological response modifiers are increasingly impacting the practice and cost of medical care. The use of hematopoietic growth factors may enable significant dose intensification of most commonly used chemotherapy regimens and may also facilitate the performance of outpatient-based bone marrow and peripheral blood stem cell transplantation.[37,38] The length of hospital stay and, hence, the cost for patients admitted to the hospital for neutropenic fever following chemotherapy may also be reduced in some patient groups with growth factor support.[39-41] EPO has decreased the need for blood transfusions and exposure to homologous blood in a number of disease states.[42-45] The expense of these growth factors and therapeutic cytokines and the toxicities of some of them have encouraged a search for ways to optimize further the desired effects and to minimize undesired ones. The recent discovery that hematopoietic growth factors and biological response modifiers are highly circadian stage dependent in their toxicities and efficacies points to one strategy by which protein drug efficacy may be optimized.

Due to the expense of these proteins, it would clearly be an advantage if a similar therapeutic effect could be achieved with a smaller dose administered at an optimal circadian time. In addition, similar to optimal circadian timing of chemotherapy drugs, diminishing the toxicity of proteins, such as TNF, interferon, and IL-2, by optimal timing is also a desirable goal. Let us now examine each of these agents in turn with respect to their activity and to the data generated thus far in chronobiological studies.

2.10.1 ERYTHROPOIETIN

EPO is a protein hormone produced by the kidney, the function of which is to stimulate bone marrow erythroid precursors to differentiate and produce mature erythrocytes. Clinical physiological studies have demonstrated that there is a prominent and reproducible circadian variation in the serum concentration of EPO. Diurnal serum EPO concentrations vary two- to threefold within the normal range with peak values near sleep onset.[46,47] A series of studies have reported the efficacy of subcutaneous recombinant human EPO given to normal female CD_2F_1 mice varies dependent upon the time of day of its administration. The blood reticulocyte response to a single circadian time dose of EPO varied almost sevenfold with maximal response around sleep onset.[48,49] After serial, circadian-timed dosing of EPO, the increment in red cell mass and the rapidity of the erythropoietic response was also maximal when administered around sleep onset.[50] Studies in tumor-bearing, anemic C_3HeB/FeJ female mice also demonstrated that the circadian-dependent efficacy of EPO was not abolished by the presence of a tumor.[51]

Based on these preclinical results, a clinical trial comparing different times of day of EPO administration in dialysis patients has been initiated. The final results of these trials are eagerly anticipated, as they may have a significant impact on the efficacy of EPO, possible dosing requirements, and therefore costs of therapy. Clinical circadian-timed EPO trials will also need to be carried out in patients with neoplastic disease and acquired immune deficiency syndrome-related anemia.

2.10.2 GRANULOCYTE COLONY-STIMULATING FACTOR

The ability of recombinant human G-CSF to increase the white blood cell and neutrophil concentrations in normal C_3HeB/FeJ mice has been examined as a function of the time of day of administration.[52] The efficacy of G-CSF to increase blood neutrophil concentrations was significantly greater when given in late activity than other times of the day. G-CSF can also activate mature granulocyte cell functions with *in vivo* antitumor activity reported in some animal tumor models.[53] Antitumor activity was also demonstrable in C_3HeB/FeJ mice with a transplantable mammary tumor. This occurred, however, only when G-CSF was administered in late activity coincident with the maximal effect on peripheral blood neutrophil numbers. No antitumor activity was seen when G-CSF was administered in the sleep phase. Human studies to examine the effect of time of day of G-CSF administration on efficacy of myeloid recovery after chemotherapy or stem cell blood mobilization appear warranted.

2.10.3 INTERLEUKIN-2

The mechanisms of antitumor action of biological response modifiers such as IL-2 are not well understood. Many different activities have been proposed, including a direct toxic effect on tumor cells and indirect effects on the host immune system and tumor support mechanisms.[54-57] The circadian dependence of human recombinant administration IL-2 host toxicity, immune effects, and antitumor effects have been defined in mice and rats. Toxicity of IL-2 measured by lethality and serum corticosterone response was lowest when IL-2 was given to mice in mid to late activity.[58] Immune cell effects, including increase in spleen size and increase in spleen Lyt 5.2 (natural killer) cells, were greatest when IL-2 was administered in early activity span.[59]

The circadian dependence of the antitumor activity of IL-2 has been studied in several *in vivo* tumor models. When IL-2 is administered by a 14-day continuous hepatic artery infusion in rats with transplanted hepatic tumors, a strong time-of-day-dependent liver toxicity was noted. Minimal hepatic toxicity and the maximum tolerated dose was seen when the peak dose of IL-2 was given in late sleep phase. Significantly greater liver toxicity and mortality was seen when IL-2 was given as a flat 24-h infusion with no circadian weighting of the dose.[60] Antitumor activity of IL-2 in this study against a transplanted hepatoma was significantly greater when the dose was weighted in late sleep compared with a flat continuous infusion. It was encouraging that the least-toxic schedule also held the greatest antitumor efficacy.

An additional circadian antitumor study of IL-2 in BALB/c mice bearing a subcutaneous sarcoma has been reported.[61] After seven daily subcutaneous injections of IL-2 at a distant site, a marked difference in tumor modulation was observed with the time of day of IL-2 administration. When IL-2 was administered in late sleep, significant inhibition of tumor size and growth rate was seen.[61] When IL-2 was administered in mid activity, not only was inhibition of tumor size not seen, but an actual marked increase in tumor size and growth rate was observed. The optimal antitumor activity resulting from late sleep administration of subcutaneous IL-2 is consistent with the findings of Kemeny et al.[60]

These preclinical animal data lead one to believe that, in fact, there could be a significant clinical difference in tumor response and severity of toxicity depending upon the circadian time of IL-2 administration. The clinical antitumor utility of IL-2 has been severely limited by low response rates and very significant toxicities. Clinical studies of IL-2 timing within the day should be explored as a strategy to optimize the desired effects while minimizing toxicities.

2.10.4 TUMOR NECROSIS FACTOR-A

Preclinical studies in mice have reported very large circadian-dependent differences in both endotoxin-induced lethality[60,62,63] and TNF-induced lethality.[64,65] The probability of dying from endotoxin or TNF varied up to ninefold depending on the time of day of its administration. Maximum survival occurred after administration of endotoxin or TNF in mid sleep. Antitumor response rates with TNF in humans have been disappointingly low and achieved at doses causing near shocklike syndrome or symptoms. The modulation in lethal toxicity by circadian timing in preclinical studies should be further pursued in optimizing the dose intensity and possibly the antitumor activity of this very toxic cytokine in humans.

2.10.5 INTERFERONS

In the last decade, the use of interferons has become commonplace in clinical hematology and oncology. Interferon is now utilized in hematologic malignancies, such as hairy cell leukemia, multiple myeloma, chronic myelogenous leukemia, and lymphoma, and in solid tumors, such as Kaposi's sarcoma, melanoma, RCC, and colon cancer.[66,67] Owing to limited single-agent activity, interferon is often used in combination with standard anticancer agents, either concomitantly or sequentially. Significant side effects of interferon, including malaise, nausea, fever, and hematologic and neurological toxicity, limit the delivery of adequate doses and patient compliance. Modulation of toxicities would increase compliance and dose intensity. The antitumor activities of interferons may occur through direct cytostatic effects on tumor cells and/or through antiangiogenic and immunodulatory effects of these cytokines.

The responsiveness of lymphoid cells to *in vitro* stimulation by interferon α[68] and γ[69] both vary with the circadian time of procurement of donor blood cells. Several murine studies have defined that many interferon-mediated effects *in vivo* are also circadian time dependent. The myelotoxicity of interferon, defined by depression in white blood cell counts and marrow myeloid colony numbers, was least when interferon α was given around sleep onset and least when interferon γ was administered in mid activity.[70,71] Anecdotal clinical reports have also claimed increased patient tolerance of interferon α with evening administration.[72] A Phase I clinical trial of ten patients with metastatic melanoma or RCC has been reported using continuous infusion interferon α with a circadian-shaped weighted administration.[73] Each course consisted of a 21-day intravenous circadian-shaped administration of interferon-α with the majority of the dose given between 2:00 p.m. and 10:00 p.m., and minimal dose between 6:00 a.m. and 10:00 a.m. The investigators initiated the trial at 15 million units/m²/day with escalation to 20 million units/m²/day. The toxicity of this circadian-shaped interferon infusion was compared with other historical trials of infusional interferon α where 1 to 7 million units/m²/day was given for 6 weeks[74] or 30 million units/m²/day was given for 5 days.[75] The usual toxicities of fatigue, flulike illness, bone marrow suppression, and somnolence were noted in the circadian-weighted infusion. However, when compared with the earlier studies, these symptoms appeared to be less marked, and the circadian infusion subsequently permitted the interferon to be given in a more dose-intensive fashion. No direct comparison in a prospective randomized trial has yet been performed. Antitumor activity of interferon-α and interferon-γ has been demonstrated to vary with the circadian time of administration in a murine tumor model.[76]

2.10.6 ADRENOCORTICOTROPIN

Adrenocorticosteroids are well known to exhibit a circadian variation in plasma concentration, being lowest in late activity and highest just around awakening. The administration of exogenous corticosteroids has a varying ability to perturb the natural rhythms depending upon the dose used and the circadian schedule employed. Divided-dose steroids markedly suppress normal adrenal function while every-other-day single-dose or single-morning-dose steroids do not disrupt the normal circadian corticosteroid pattern and do not markedly suppress the hypothalamus–adrenal axis almost regardless of dose.

It is not known whether or not the timing of administration of corticosteroids is important for their antitumor activity, but timing is critical to their use and appears to be much more so when they are administered as antiemetics prior to the administration of conventional chemotherapeutic agents. The reasons for concern include the fact that endogenous corticosterone markedly alters the ability of an animal to tolerate chemotherapy. Interfering with levels of endogenous corticosterones by exogenous administration changes the ability of the animal to withstand the toxicity of the chemotherapy and could also theoretically increase the resistance of a tumor to its effects. In corroboration of these concepts, investigators found that administration of dexamethasone to animals for 10 days prior to giving them methotrexate suppressed their endogenous corticosterone levels, and all animals subsequently died within 5 days of methotrexate administration.[77] In animals receiving corticosterone, the toxicity was significantly less than in those receiving dexamethasone or placebo. As the methotrexate was administered at one of multiple times during the circadian cycle in each group of animals, it was interesting to note that the time of maximal toxicity was found to be in the late activity span.

When administered prior to cyclophosphamide in Erlich ascites carcinoma–bearing female mice, exogenous corticosteroids markedly decreased the antitumor effects of the chemotherapy.[78,79] Lévi et al.[80] found that the administration of ACTH 24 h. before doxorubicin raised protective levels of GSH to the maximum circadian level in a variety of murine tissues, which subsequently protected these tissues from toxicity. As has been indicated before, the GSH–GSSG levels as well as their ability to be raised by ACTH vary significantly on a circadian basis.

It is felt that corticosteroids may interfere with the uptake of methotrexate by lymphoblastoid cells. Interestingly, a report by Rivard et al.[81] indicates that children with lymphoblastic leukemia had improved survival when maintenance chemotherapy, consisting of daily 6-mercaptopurine and weekly methotrexate, was administered in the evening hours, coinciding with the lowest daily levels of endogenous corticosteroids.

It is tempting to hypothesize that it may be possible to modulate the internal circadian time structure by the exogenous administration of agents such as corticosteroids or melatonin. This has been tested in transatlantic pilots, and is reported to ameliorate the severity of jet lag.[82] In addition, some interesting effects have been noted in rats given both corticosteroids and melatonin, which theoretically extends the "dark" phase in photoperiodic species.[83] This exciting area of chronobiotic therapy requires further exploration. This exploration could potentially enable patients to be treated at a much more precise chronobiological time by prospectively synchronizing internal time clocks in a predictable fashion.

2.11 TIMED DELIVERY OF THERAPEUTIC AGENTS

Having established that there is an optimal chronobiological time for the delivery of most cancer chemotherapeutic agents, the next question is the optimal method of administration. Clearly, if the agents to be administered are given by a bolus injection, then simply planning the administration at the optimal chronotherapeutic time is straightforward. The issue becomes somewhat more complex, however, when the drug or biological response modifier is delivered by a continuous infusion over a prolonged period. In this case, not only will adequate venous or arterial access be important, but there is also a need for a reliable, programmable delivery device which is able to administer the drug according to a predetermined optimal chronotherapeutic schedule. In addition, the physical–chemical properties of the delivered agent and the potential interaction between the agent and the surfaces of the pumping device and the connecting tubing will need to be understood and incorporated into the planning of the administration.[84-87]

2.11.1 DEVICES

The selection of the optimal device to deliver the agent of choice will depend upon the nature of the agent being delivered, the intended route of administration, the anticipated duration of infusion, the life expectancy of the patient, and the complexity of the program. Two broad categories of pump are now available: the totally implantable pump and the portable external pump connected to the patient by a subcutaneous venous or arterial access device.[88-91]

2.11.1.1 Implantable Pumps

The most readily available example of this type of pump is the SynchroMed® by Medtronic. This is a totally implanted infusion device which is programmable in time so that a variety of alternative circadian infusion schedules is possible. This pump has been used for both intravenous and intra-arterial drug administration and has proved to be effective and reliable. The advantages of a totally implanted pump such as this are (1) convenience for the patient, as there is no external tubing or external pump which needs to be carried about; (2) the low risk of infection because of the self-contained nature of the pump; (3) cost of the device (although the device is expensive, a study comparing an implantable pump with externally available devices has concluded that the implantable pump is advantageous if the patient survives for a long enough period of time[92]); and (4) no tampering with, or inadvertent damage to, the pump is possible because of its internal location. The disadvantages are (1) a surgical procedure is required for implantation of the pump; (2) the cost of the pump can be a significant factor if the patient survives for a short period of time; (3) the pump is non-reusable and, when the patient dies, the pump is lost to further use; (4) the programming of the pump requires a special external wand and is fairly complex, requiring specialized training. In addition, the pump must always have fluid in its reservoir and needs to be filled with saline during the time that chemotherapy is not administered. The patient also has to be physically present to alter the programming. This means that the patient cannot switch the pump off should a malfunction occur. (5) Multiple agents in a complex chronotherapeutic regimen cannot be administered simultaneously with these pumps.

2.11.1.2 Portable External Pumps

Examples of this type of pump include the Strato Pump (no longer available), the Vivus 2000® and 4000® pumps by Iflow, the Panomate® pump by Disetronic, the Intelliject® pump by Intelligent Medicine, the Minimed® pump by Minimed Technologies, and the CADD-Plus® or the CADD-TPN® pump by Pharmacia-Deltec. As can be seen from this listing, there are many more external portable pumps than implantable devices.[88,89] The advantages of an external pump include the following: (1) the volume of infused solution is very flexible, with the smallest pump containing 3 ml and the larger pumps, using an external reservoir, containing any volume desired; (2) multiple agents may be administered simultaneously by some of these pumps, such as the Intelliject and the Vivus pumps, and this allows a complex, multiagent chronobiological program; (3) the pumps are all reusable and, should the patient die or fail to respond to the therapy, the pump may be reused in an alternative program or in a different patient; (4) the pumps are programmed by an external device but may be switched off by the patient in the event of untoward effects; (5) when the pump is not in use, it is disconnected from the venous access device, usually a subcutaneous port such as an Infusaport®, and the patient is then totally free of any devices or the need for continuous filling of the pump; and, finally, (6) because the pumps are reusable, their cost is considerably less than a totally implantable pump unless used for a prolonged period when the costs of nursing visits and administration may exceed that of a totally implantable device. The disadvantages of these pumps include (1) a venous or arterial access device needs to be placed; (2) infectious risk is greater because of the external nature of the pump and the associated tubing and transcutaneous access; (3) patient tampering or damage is possible; and (4) weight and inconvenience of carrying the portable device, which is particularly germane in the case of elderly or frail patients.

As can be seen from the above description, the most suitable pump for a given application must be determined. Virtually any chronotherapeutic program is possible by the choice of the correct device, which may clearly be very well managed by many home health care agencies and thus limit the need for multiple visits to the primary treatment center.

2.11.2 PROBLEMS

Unfortunately, as fluids containing therapeutic agents have both physical and chemical properties, the delivery of such fluids is not always simple. Among the devices listed above, the actual pumping mechanism varies. This may consist of either a linear or rotary peristaltic device, a cassette device, a gear-actuated syringe infusion, or a motor-driven screw. These each have inherent advantages and disadvantages.

The peristaltic devices apply shear forces upon the administered agent, which is clearly detrimental if this happens to be a protein or a peptide such as a biological response modifier. This is not a problem when the agent is a simple chemotherapeutic drug. Syringe devices, on the other hand, do not apply shear force to the agent and therefore are suitable for proteins and peptides. However, they are severely limited by their small volume.

A further major problem associated with continuous infusion delivery devices is the interaction between the delivered drug and the surface of the device and its associated tubing. This is a particularly pronounced problem for the protein and peptide agents, such as the biological response modifiers. This problem is well recognized and has been described for many common pharmacological agents such as benzodiazopenes, nitroglycerin, and insulin.[85] Not only can drugs adhere to the artificial surfaces, and therefore be lost to the patient, but they may also be structurally altered by this interaction and lose biological activity despite being administered.[84,86,87,89]

A very elegant demonstration of these phenomena has been reported for IL-2.[90] Continuous delivery of IL-2 at 37 °C over a 24-h period resulted in a 20 to 30% reduction in the ultimate concentration of delivered IL-2 relative to the initial concentration. There was a significant initial drop with subsequent increase to an equilibrium state, undoubtedly owing to saturation of the binding sites in the tubing. In addition, the biological activity of the IL-2 was further decreased by almost 90% during flow through a medical-grade silicone catheter, because of conformational changes in the protein structure. These changes resulted from momentary contact with the surface and/or the partially denatured IL-2 adsorbed to that surface.

Clearly, then, any loss in delivered biological activity compared with the projected activity, based on initial concentration and flow rate, can result in a gross underestimate of the efficacy and potency of a delivered agent. Many different strategies have been adopted in an attempt to modify these effects, including the stabilization of the protein solution using human serum albumin, the provision of an optimal pH and osmotic pressure, and the use of substances such as surfactants and antioxidants.[87,89] This can lead to a marked improvement in the ultimate delivered dose of an agent. A good example, recently demonstrated, is the abrogation of the severe loss of recombinant TNF when administered by burette-type administration sets, by the simple addition of 0.25% albumin.[84] This results in a diminution of lost activity from 94 to 2%. It is important, therefore, for any clinician planning to administer an agent, particularly a protein or peptide, by continuous infusion through a constant delivery device to determine whether or not there will be any protein or peptide surface interaction and, if so, to determine its nature and the optimal method for abrogating this effect. In this way, significant errors in administration will be avoided.

In the future, more-sophisticated devices will be available, which will not only be programmable but which may respond via sensors to internal biorhythms.[88,91,93-95] These may include devices that deliver drugs through a transdermal route and utilize either electric current or ultrasound waves to drive the agent through the skin. Alternatively, magnets may be used to vary the release of drugs from implanted devices in an extremely accurate and controllable fashion.[96]

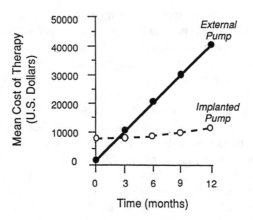

FIGURE 2.7   Cost of treatment with external and implanted pumps.

2.12   COSTS OF INFUSIONAL TREATMENT

Not so long ago, if long-term infusional therapy was given, it was administered only in the inpatient setting. The cost of days, weeks, or months of continuous infusion chemotherapy were, therefore, extremely high. This was true whether the therapy was administered systemically or locally; intravenously or intra-arterially. The development of long-term venous access devices (first transcutaneous and, later, implanted) and the development of wearable single-rate pumps (and, later, programmable drug pumps) have made it possible to deliver infusional chemotherapy in an entirely outpatient setting. Other advances have led to the development of further generations of multiple-channel and flexibly programmable pumps that can deliver temporally precise patterns of chemotherapy. These facts and products have resulted in the rapid growth of a new home care industry. The health care delivery system benefits from relatively lower costs, and the patients benefit from the lower toxicity of long-term infusion and from being at home. The value of these additions to the quality of a cancer patient's life is hard to overestimate.

Infusional home care managed by professional home care operations is less expensive than hospitalizing the patient. These costs have, however, escalated substantially in the past years. The physician who writes the orders assumes all medical and most legal responsibilities, while home care networks independently set and collect the fees associated with this care. This has resulted in a substantial shift of revenue from the hospital and, to a lesser extent, from the physician's office to the home care company.

It would initially appear that placement of a $6000 programmable implanted drug delivery system is more expensive than treatment with a wearable programmable pump. We have, however, discovered that this is not the case. Figure 2.7 demonstrates that if the patient receiving single-agent infusional therapy receives treatment for longer than 3 months, it is substantially less expensive to implant a programmable device than it is to deliver this therapy using a wearable pump. If the patient lives on therapy 6 months, it is almost twice as expensive to use a wearable pump. More than 95% of our patients are on therapy for at least 3 months, and more than 80% receive this infusional therapy for at least 6 months. Responders often receive therapy for more than 2 years.

The major difference in cost is more related to where the fees go, rather than how much the therapy costs the health care system. If a large home care company is used, the majority of the costs go to that company. If an implantable device is used, the major initial costs are for the device and the implantation procedure, while all follow-up costs go to covering the physician's expenses for management of the patient. No costs go to a separate home care management company.

2.13 ECONOMIC PRESSURE OF GOVERNMENTAL ORIGIN FOR THE USE OF AUTOMATIC DRUG DELIVERY SYSTEMS

The latest, effective government attempt to decrease the costs of medical care mitigates strongly against inpatient medical evaluation and therapy. Whereas 2 years ago most cancer therapy was given in the hospital, currently fewer patients are admitted for inpatient treatment. While the outpatient clinic is the major site of cancer therapy, these clinics are not optimally configured to give complex time-oriented, multiday, multidose, or even multidrug therapy. On the other hand, it is the opinion of many oncologists that the most effective anticancer regimens are becoming more complex, not simpler. If patients are to receive the benefit, economically, of the latest and most effective multidrug, multiday, multidose, and time-specified bolus and infusional treatments, a way must be devised. Programmed automatic drug delivery devices obviously provide the method, both in principle and in practice.

Many complex protocols for the treatment of a variety of cancers could be moved from the inpatient to the outpatient setting by the intelligent use of these kinds of devices. The patient's desire for the best available treatment will result in utilization of ever more complex protocols, while government and private sector pressure will demand widespread use of such instruments to reduce the cost of responding to these demands.

Pharmacy-related costs are also a sizable component of inpatient and outpatient treatment cost. The use of automatic drug delivery systems and prepackaged drug regimens can markedly reduce these costs as well.

2.14 INDUSTRIAL-BASED ECONOMIC PRESSURE

The scientific drought, reflected by the lack of promising new anticancer drugs combined with the length of time required to gain FDA approval for new drugs, has resulted in tremendous pressure on large pharmaceutical firms producing anticancer drugs. At the same time, the lack of exciting, new, even "tarnished silver bullets," has many physicians and cooperative clinical research groups thinking about new ways to give old drugs. These "old drugs" are not proprietary.

If new therapies and new drugs are ever to develop, the huge costs of research, development, marketing, and jumping through the required regulatory hoops must be paid. One approach to this is a natural tripartite alliance among drug makers, device manufacturers, and clinical research laboratories to develop regimens which can be protected by meaningful method patents or unique technological know-how. Optimal complex therapeutic regimens developed at research centers, using research funds supplied by both device and drug manufacturers, may be protected by method patents, trade secrets, limited hardware/software drug formulation–limited compatibility, patents upon hardware and software, and by single-device-compatible drug packaging. This would result in nonproprietary drugs regaining a proprietary advantage. This approach will result in the most advanced and complex protocols being widely available to patients largely in the outpatient setting. It will also result in the cost accounting of clinical research and an appropriate return to device and drug manufacturers for funding the research that is necessary to develop these regimens and devices. In addition, favorable patent and tax treatment for drug companies may also be available for developing new indications for nonproprietary "orphan" drugs.

While these strategies for protocol development and funding do not obviate the need for the discovery of new and better anticancer drugs, any practicing oncologist will soon admit that there may be better and worse ways to use the currently available drugs, and that there is likely to be some return for the cancer patient by moving in this direction.

2.15 MEDICAL PRESSURES FOR THE USE OF AUTOMATIC PROGRAMMABLE DRUG DELIVERY DEVICES

The medical community will insist on the availability of such devices, because their proper use will allow the simpler, easier administration of the optimal disease-related complex protocols; protocols that are more effective than current ones. No physician will adopt the use of a device that will complicate and increase the cost of the physician's practice by requiring more of the physician's time or his or her nurse's time. However, these devices will ultimately be put together in such a way as to require less time and less attention than standard methods of giving therapy (they will be very simple, operationally). Shell programs and premixed, prepackaged hardware and/or software specific drug regimens, combined with long-term parenteral access catheters, will ultimately make delivery of complex regimens simpler than giving weekly intravenous 5-FU (the simplest, most widely used anticancer regimen).

2.16 MEDICAL CONSUMER (PATIENT) PRESSURE

The "patient as consumer" will exert substantial pressure. The oversupply of physicians of all varieties has resulted in a profound and increasing competition for patients. This has put these physicians in a position of needing to deliver the best care, in order to maintain their patient base and income. When patients become aware of the advantages of automatic drug delivery systems, they will demand them and the physician will supply this demand.

2.17 MEDICAL ACCURACY

Errors of dosage and errors of drug timing and sequence can be diminished by the employment of simple-to-use, smart devices. The frequency of inpatient and outpatient therapeutic errors is not something which is discussed much, but something about which each physician, nurse, and pharmacist is acutely aware. Errors do occur. Sometimes they result in insignificant consequences, and sometimes in catastrophic consequences. At a typical hospital, there are 11 steps between the writing of an intravenous medication order and its actual delivery. At each juncture, an error of several varieties is possible. New hardware, software, and premixed drug modules can result in decreasing the possibilities for error. The advantages of this in economic and medical terms may be difficult to overestimate.

2.18 SCIENTIFIC PRESSURES

2.18.1 Lack of Curative Regimens

The need for new ideas relevant to the treatment, control, and cure of the common cancers is stimulating reevaluation of drug scheduling, combinations, routes, and timings. Natural genetically engineered biological substances open up new therapeutic avenues and new hope for these common cancers. The circadian timing, sequence, and interval among doses, agents, or cycle of these agents are likely, however, to be even more critical than for cytotoxics. The availability of automatic programmable drug delivery devices opens new vistas of relevant and interesting science that will impact upon cancer control and cure.

2.18.2 Protocol Compliance

National Cooperative Study Group protocol compliance can be substantially improved by the intelligent use of these devices. Clinical research trial sponsors, whether federal or private, can easily assure that common research done in several centers is truly comparable. The use of these systems will markedly facilitate and assure comparability across institutions.

2.18.3 The Intelligent Use of Biological Therapy

While it has been adequately demonstrated that the therapeutic ratio of toxicity of anticancer drugs is dependent to a large extent upon the timing of drug delivery (relative to circadian time, time between doses, and drug sequence), these variables are much more relevant to the effective use of biological response modifiers. The time of day when interferons, leukotrienes, tumor necrosis factors, IL-2, LAK cells, growth factors, or monoclonal antibodies are given — relative to the patient's circadian cycle, repeat dosages, their sequences vis à vis one another, and standard cytotoxic treatment — ultimately will determine how effective these approaches are. In a series of chronotoxicological experiments recently completed at the University of Minnesota, the lethal toxicity of human recombinant TNF has been demonstrated to be reproducibly variable according to when in the day it is given to mice. This time-dependent difference in lethal toxicity is tenfold.

The standard Phase I and Phase II approaches to the study of biological agents will not adequately define their activity or even the relevant toxicities of these agents, even though they have profound biological effects in picogram quantities at the level of the cell. The relationship between host and tumor is elegantly and temporally complex. Giving milligram quantities of biologicals without regard to this complexity will only result in great expense, great toxicity, and, finally, great frustration. The availability of instruments able to stipulate sequence, interval, circadian stage, and infradian pattern of immune modulation is a *sine qua non* to optimal biotherapy.

Programmable implanted and wearable devices and biocompatible catheters also raise the possibility of local or regional immunomodulation. This temporal and spatial optimization may eliminate the need to expose the patient systemically, diminishing or eliminating many of the toxicities of these biological anticancer agents.

2.19 HOW THESE DRUG DELIVERY SYSTEMS WILL ULTIMATELY BE USED

Automatic, programmable, implanted, wearable, and bedside systems will have uses in virtually every specialty of modern medicine and surgery. Initially, open-loop and, subsequently, closed-loop multiple drug systems will pervade medical practice.

Modern oncology will demand circadian timing–stipulated, multidrug regimens, biological therapies, and hybrid chemobiotherapies. Each of these types of therapy will not only stipulate time of day of each dose, but how many hours or days between repeat cycles, and the order in which the agents or patterns of agents are to be used. Polypharmacy is the rule in oncology, making multiple reservoir systems very useful. Implantable systems will be used for locoregional therapy, for quasi-continuous systemic cell cycle synchronization, and for long-term immune modulation. These systems will be complemented by the use of extracorporeal devices for short-term therapy in the same patients.

Protocol design will no longer be constrained by questions of protocol compliance. National cooperative groups and Cooperative Clinical Oncology Programs (C-COPs) will be able to test and apply complex basic findings effectively to the more immediate benefit of the patient with cancer.

Endocrinology will someday rely upon implanted, closed-loop, artificial hypothalamus, pituitary, adrenal, and pancreas technologies. In the interim, many advances will be made possible by simple, closed-loop systems. Right now, ultradian (high-frequency) and circadian-patterned therapy is essential in treating fertility and growth problems, and it will soon be required to alleviate sleep and emotional disorders.

Effective biotherapy will require complex administration of a wide variety of drugs and biologicals. Their application in rheumatology, transplantation, cancer therapy, and treatment of immunodeficiency syndromes (including AIDS) will be expedited by these kinds of delivery systems. In hematology, desferoxamine chelation treatment of iron overload may be improved by automatic delivery systems.

Cardiologists and nephrologists treating arrhythmias or hypertension soon will be assisted by closed-loop automatic systems, in which these new technologies will "sense" the events that prompt therapeutic interventions. Even before this, however, programmed, circadian-modified, transcutaneous, or intravenous delivery of nitroglycerin, nitroprusside, dopamine, xylocaine, and other drugs may make sense.

Rheumatologists, allergists, and pulmonary doctors may use anti-inflammatory agents and bronchodilators that are best given with careful consideration to their circadian timing with the use of automatic programmable devices. Gastroenterologists, meanwhile, will use H-2 blocking agents which have been prepared to be bioavailable at the time of day associated with highest basal and stimulated acid secretion (2 to 4 a.m.).

Intensive care unit acute care medicine may be the first place where polypharmacy will be used in a closed-loop manner, administering diverse drugs to patients with multiple organ failure, according to the physiological–biochemical signals fed to the device directly from the patients' monitoring devices. These and many other applications will be generated as these devices mature, become easier to use, and are expanded to do more, more simply.

2.20   THE PRACTICE OF MEDICINE AND CHRONOBIOLOGY

The adoption of "intelligent" automatic, programmable, drug delivery devices will make medicine both intrinsically more complex and extrinsically more simple. It will make delivery of complex drug and biological regimens safer, less error prone, and less expensive. The therapy of serious diseases will be more uniform. Protocols developed in university centers and by clinical research groups will be widely available to all medical practitioners and, once instituted, will be carried out more exactly. Better medicine will ultimately be more widely available to more patients.

The clinical research to establish these protocols should be funded by collaboration among government, industry, and academics. The pressure to market new drugs may decrease and might well be replaced by a more rational pressure to discover and effectively protect the best way of giving drugs. A wide variety of devices and competing protocols will keep each system and protocol cost-effective, and this competition will both assure a return on investment and hold down costs. This cost accounting of clinical applications research will result in less-expensive medical care.

Finally, the adoption of programmed automatic drug delivery will bring attention to temporal chronobiological questions which have been, until now, unanswerable. This attention will turn chronobiology into what it truly is — a multidimensional and dynamic perspective on life science. This medical movement toward temporal considerations will abolish the separate science of chronobiology and ultimately make all biologists and physicians chronobiologists.

REFERENCES

1. Haus, E., Halberg, .F, Scheving, L. et al., Increased tolerance of mice to arabinosyl-cytosine given on schedule adjusted to circadian system. *Science* 1972; 177:80–82.
2. Scheving, L.E., Haus, E., Kuhl, J.F.W. et al., Close reproduction by different laboratories of characteristics of circadian rhythm in 1-β-D-arabinfuranosylcytosine. *Cancer Res.* 1976; 36:1133–1137.
3. Freireich, E., Ara-C; a twenty year update. *J. Clin. Oncol.* 1987; 5:523–524.
4. Hrushesky, W.J.M., Circadian timing of cancer chemotherapy. *Science* 1985; 228:73–75.
5. Lévi, F., Mechkouri, M., Roulon, A. et al., Circadian rhythm in tolerance of mice for the new anthracycline analog 4′-tetrahydropyranyladriamycin (THP). *Eur. J. Cancer Clin. Oncol.* 1985; 121:1245–1251.
6. Mormont, M.C., Roemeling, R.V., Sothern, R.B. et al., Circadian rhythm and seasonal dependence in the toxicological response of mice to epirubicin. *Invest. New Drugs* 1988; 6:273–283.
7. Scheving, L.E., Burns, R., Pauly, J.E., Halberg, F., Haus, E., Survival and care of leukemic mice after circadian optimization of treatment with cyclophosphamide and 1-β-D-arabinofuranosylcytosine. *Cancer Res.* 1977; 37:3648–3655.
8. Sothern, R.B., Levi, F., Haus, E., Halberg, F., Hrushesky, W.J.M., Doxorubicin-cisplatin control of a murine plasmacytoma depends upon circadian stage of treatment. *J. Natl. Cancer Inst.* 1988; 80:1232–1237.
9. Hrushesky, W.J.M., The clinical application of chronobiology to oncology. *Am. J. Anat.* 1983; 168:519–542.
10. Hrushesky, W.J.M., von Roemeling, R., Sothern, B., Circadian chronotherapy: from animal experiments to human cancer chemotherapy. In Lemmer B, Ed. *Chronopharmacology: Cellular and Biochemical Interactions.* New York: Marcel Dekker, 1989:439–473.
11. Popovic, P., Popovic, V., Baughman, J., Circadian rhythm and 5-fluorouracil toxicity in C_3H mice. *Biomed. Thermol.* 1982; 25:185–187.
12. Burns, R.E., Beland, S.S., Effect of biological time on the determination of the LD50 of 5-fluorouracil in mice. *Pharmacology* 1984; 28:296–300.
13. Peters, G.J., Van Dijk, J., Nadal, J.C., Van Groeningen, C.J., Lankelman, J., Pinedo, H.M., Diurnal variation in the therapeutic efficacy of 5-fluorouracil against murine colon cancer. *In Vivo* 1987; 1:112–118.
14. Gonzalez, R.B., Sothern, R.B., Thatcher, G., Nguyen, N., Hrushesky, W.J.M., Substantial difference in timing of murine circadian susceptibility to 5-fluorouracil and FUDR. *Proc. Am. Assoc. Can. Res.* 1989; 30:2452a.
15. von Roemeling, R., Hrushesky, W., Circadian FUDR infusion pattern determines its therapeutic index. *J. Natl. Cancer Inst.* 1990; 82:386–393.
16. von Roemeling, R., Hrushesky, W.J.M., Circadian patterning of continuous floxuridine infusion reduces toxicity and allows higher dose intensity in patients with widespread cancer. *J. Clin. Oncol.* 1989; 7:1710–1719.
17. Hrushesky, W.J.M., von Roemeling, R., Lanning, R.M., Rabatin, J.T., Circadian-shaped infusion of floxuridine for progressive metastatic renal cell carcinoma. *J. Clin. Oncol.* 1990; 8:1504–1513.
18. von Roemeling, R., Hrushesky, W.J.M., The advantage of circadian shaping of fluorpyrimidine infusions. In Lokich, J.L., Ed. *Cancer Chemotherapy by Infusion.* Chicago: Precept Press, 1990:619–646.

19. Wesen, C., Hrushesky, W.J.M., Roemeling, R.V., Lanning, R., Rabatin, J., Grage, T., Circadian modification of intra-arterial 5-fluoro-2'-deoxyuridine infusion rate reduces its toxicity and permits higher dose intensity. *J. Infus. Chemother.* 1992; 2:69–75.

20. Lévi, F., Soussan, A., Adam, R., Programmable-in-time pumps for chronotherapy of patients with colorectal cancer with 5-day circadian-modulated venous infusion of 5-fluorouracil (CVI-5FUra), *Proc. ASCO,* 1989. Vol. Abstr. #429.

21. Petit, E., Milano, G., Levi, F., Thyss, A., Bailleul, F., Schneider, M., Circadian rhythm-varying plasma concentration of 5-fluorouracil during a five day continuous infusion at a constant rate in cancer patients. *Cancer Res.* 1988; 48:1676–1679.

22. Harris, B., Song, R., Soong, S.-J., Diasio, R., Comparison of short-term and continuous chemotherapy (mitozantrone) for advanced breast cancer. *Cancer Res.* 1990; 48:197–201.

23. Tuchman, M., Stoeckeler, J., Kiang, D., O'Dea, R., Ramnaraine, M., Mirkin, B., Sources of variability of dehydropyrimidine dehydogenase (DPD) activity in human blood mononuclear cells. *N. Engl. J. Med.* 1983; 313:245–249.

24. Diasio, R.B., Beavers, T.L., Carpenter, J.T., Familial deficiency of dihydropyrimidine dehydrogenase. Biochemical basis for familial pyrimidinemia and severe 5-fluorouracil-induced toxicity. *J. Clin. Invest.* 1988; 81:47–51.

25. Tuchman, M., von Roemeling, R., Lanning, R., Sothern, R.B., Hrushesky, W.J.M., Sources of variability of dihydropyrimidine dehydrogenase (DPD) activity in human blood mononuclear cells. *Annu. Rev. Chronopharmacol.* 1988; 5:399–402.

26. Harris, B.E., Song, R., Soong, S., Diasio, R.B., Circadian variation of 5-fluorouracil catabolism in isolated perfused rat liver. *Cancer Res.* 1989; 49:6610–6614.

27. von Roemeling, R., Fukuda, E., Fudin, J. et al., Are FUDR pharmacokinetics circadian stage dependent? *Proc. AACR* 1989:2345.

28. el Kouni, M.H., Naguib, F.M.N., Cha, S., Circadian rhythm of dihydrouracil dehydrogenase (DHUDase), uridine phosphorylase (UrdPase), and thymidine phosphorylase (dThdase) in mouse liver. *FASEB J.* 1989; 3:A397.

29. Scheving, L.E., Tsai, T.S., Feuers, R.J., Scheving, L.A., Cellular mechanisms involved in the action of anticancer drugs. In Lemmer B, Ed. *Chronopharmacology: Cellular and Biochemical Interactions.* New York: Marcel Dekker, 1989:317–369.

30. Scheving, L.E., Mitotic activity in the human epidermis. *Anat. Rec.* 1959; 135:7–19.

31. Mauer, A.M., Diurnal variation of proliferative activity in the human bone marrow. *Blood* 1965; 26:1–7.

32. Smaaland, R., Sletvold, O., Bjerknes, R., Lote, K., Laerum, O.D., Circadian variations of cell cycle distribution in human bone marrow. *Chronobiologia* 1987; 14:239.

33. Buchi, K.N., Rubin, N.J., Moore, J.G., Circadian cellular proliferation in human rectal mucosa. In Reinberg, A., Smolensky, M., Labrecque, G., Eds. *Annual Review of Chronopharmacology.* Vol. 5. Oxford: Pergamon Press, 1989:355.

34. Buchi, K.N., Moore, J.G., Hrushesky, W.J.M., Sothern, R.B., Rubin, N.H., Circadian rhythm of cellular proliferation in the human rectal mucosa. *Gastroenterology* 1991; 101:410–415.

35. Klevecz, R.R., Shymko, R.M., Blumenfeld, D., Braly, P.S., Circadian gating of S phase in human ovarian cancer. *Cancer Res.* 1987; 47:6267–6271.

36. Smaaland, R., Lote, K., Laerum, O., Vokac, Z., A circadian study of cell cycle distribution in non-Hodgkin lymphomas. In Reinberg, A., Smolensky, M., Labrecque, G., Eds. *Annual Review of Chronopharmacology.* Vol. 5. New York: Pergamon Press, 1989:383.

37. Nemunaitis, J., Rabinowe, S., Singer, J. et al., Recombinant granulocyte-macrophage colony-stimulating factor after autologous bone marrow transplantation for lymphoid cancer. *N. Engl. J. Med.* 1991; 324:1773.

38. Advani, R., Chao, N.J., Horning, S.J., et al. Granulocyte-macrophage colony-stimulating factor (GM-CSF) as an adjunct to autologous hemopoietic stem cell transplantation of lymphoma. *Ann. Intern. Med.* 1992; 116:183.

39. Crawford, J., Ozer, H., Stoller, R. et al., Reduction by granulocyte colony-stimulating factor of fever and neutropenia induced by chemotherapy in patients with small-cell lung cancer. *N. Engl. J. Med.* 1991; 315:164–170.

40. Pettengell, R., Gurney, H., Radford, J.A. et al., Granulocyte colony-stimulating factor to prevent dose-limiting neutropenia in non-Hodgkin's lymphoma: a randomized controlled trial. *Blood* 1992; 80:1430.

41. Trillett-Lenoir, V., Green, J.A., Manegold, C. et al., Recombinant granulocyte colony-stimulating factor reduces the infectious complications of cytotoxic chemotherapy. *Eur. J. Cancer,* 1993; 29A:319.

42. Triulzi, D.J., Vanek, K., Ryan, D.H., Blumberg, N., A clinical and immunologic study of blood transfusion and postoperative bacterial infection in spinal surgery. *Transfusion* 1992; 32:517–524.

43. Abels, R.I., Larholt, K.M., Krantz, K.D., Bryant, E.C., Recombinant human erythropoietin (r-HuEPO) for the treatment of the anemia of cancer. In Murphy, M.J., Ed. *Blood Cell Growth Factors: Their Present and Future Use in Hematology and Oncology.* Dayton: Alpha Medical Press, 1991:121–141.

44. Evans, R.W., Recombinant human erythropoietin and the quality of life of end-stage renal disease patients: a comparative analysis. *Am. J. Kidney Dis.* 1991; 27:62–70.

45. Jensen, L.S., Anersen, A.J., Christiansen, P.M. et al., Postoperative infection and natural killer cell function blood transfusion in patients undergoing elective colorectal surgery. *Br. J. Surg.* 1992; 79:513–516.

46. Wide, L., Bengtsson, C., Birgegard, G., Circadian rhythm of erythropoietin in human serum. *Br. J. Haematol.* 1989; 72:85–90.

47. Cotes, P.M., Brozovic, B., Diurnal variation of serum immunoreactive erythropoietin in normal subject. *Clin. Endocrinol.* 1982; 17:419–422.

48. Wood, P.A., Sanchez de la Peña, S., Hrushesky, W.J.M., Evidence for circadian dependency of recombinant human erythropoietin (rhEPO) response in the mouse. In Reinberg, A., Smolensky, M., Labreque, G., Eds. *Annual Review of Chronopharmacology.* Vol. 7. Oxford: Pergamon Press, 1990:173–176.

49. Wood, P.A., Vyzula, R., Hrushesky, W.J.M., Circadian hematopoietic growth factor chronotherapy. *J. Infus. Chemother.* 1993; 3:89–95.

50. Wood, P.A., Peace, D., Troha, T., Mann, G., Hrushesky, W.J.M., Efficacy of chronic erythropoietin is dependent upon the time of day of its administration. *Exp. Hematol.* 1994; 22:707.

51. Wood, P.A., Martynowicz, M., Sanchez, S., Chang, C., Hrushesky, W.J.M., Circadian erythropoietin pharmacodynamics. *Blood* 1991; 70:16a.

52. Vyzula, R., Whighton, T., Traynor, K. et al., Comparative circadian organization of the myelopoetic and unexpected oncomodulatory effects of granulocyte colony stimulating factor, Society for Research on Biological Rhythms. May 6–10, Amelia Island, FL, 1992.

53. Akaza, H., Fukushima, H., Koiso, K., Aso, Y., Enhancement of chemotherapeutic effects by recombinant human granulocyte colony-stimulating factor on implanted mouse bladder cancer cells (MBT-2). *Cancer* 1992; 69:997.

54. Alexander, R.B., Rosenberg, S.A., Tumor necrosis factor: clinical applications. In DeVita, V.T., Hellman, S., Rosenberg, S.A., Eds. *Biologic Therapy of Cancer.* Philadelphia: J.B. Lippincott, 1991:378–392.
55. Borden, E.C., Interferons: Pleiotropic cellular modulators. *Clin. Immunol. Immunopathol.,* 1992; 62:S18.
56. Frei, E., Spriggs, D., Tumor necrosis factor: still a promising agent. *J. Clin. Oncol.* 1989; 7:291–294.
57. Smith, K.A., Lowest dose interleukin-2 immunotherapy. *Blood* 1993; 81:1414–1423.
58. Lévi, F., Bourin, P., Pages, N. et al., Dosing-time of IL-2 affects both lethal and central nervous system toxicity in mice. *Proc. Am. Assoc. Cancer Res.* 1992; 33:329.
59. von Roemeling, R., DeMaria, L., Salzer, M. et al., Circadian stage dependent response to interleukin-2 in mouse spleen and bone marrow, *Annual Review of Chronopharmacology,* Vol. 7, Oxford: Pergamon Press, 1990.
60. Kemeny, M., Alava, G., Oliver, J., Improving responses in hepatoma with circadian patterned hepatic artery infusions of recombinant interleukin-2. *J. Immunother.* 1992; 12:219–223.
61. Hrushesky, W.J.M., Sánchez, S., Wood, P.A. et al., Heterogeneity of interleukin-2 therapeutic activity. *Proc. Am. Assoc. Cancer Res.* 1992; 33:300.
62. Halberg, F., Johnson, E.A., Brown, B.W., Bittner, J.J., Susceptibility rhythm to *E. coli* endotoxin and bioassay. *Proc. Soc. Exp. Biol. Med.* 1960; 103:142–144.
63. Elliot, G.T., Welty, D., Kuo, Y.D., The D-galactosamine loaded mouse and its enhanced sensitivity to lipopolysaccharide and monophosphoryl lipid A: a role for superoxide. *J. Immunol.* 1991; 10:69–74.
64. Hrushesky, W.J.M., Langevin, T., Kim, Y.J., Wood, P.A., Circadian dynamics of tumor necrosis factor-a (cachectin) lethality. *J. Exp. Med.* 1994; 180:1059–1065.
65. Langevin, T., Young, J., Walker, K., Roemeling, R., Nygaard, S., Hrushesky, W.J.M., The toxicity of tumor necrosis factor (TNF) is reproducibly different at specific times of the day. *Proc. Annu. Meeting Am. Assoc. Cancer. Res.* 1987; 28:A1580.
66. Oken, M.M., New agents for the treatment of multiple myeloma and non-Hodgkin lymphoma. *Cancer* 1992; 70:946.
67. Wadler, S., The role of interferons in the treatment of solid tumors. *Cancer* 1992; 70:4.
68. Canon, C., Levi, F., Immune system in relation to cancer. In Touitou, Y., Haus, E., Eds. *Biologic rhythms in clinical and laboratory medicine.* New York: Springer-Verlag, 1992:635–647.
69. Gatti, G., Masera, R., Cavallo, R. et al., Circadian variation of interferon-induced enhancement of human natural killer (NK) cell activity. *Cancer Detect. Prevent.* 1988; 12:431–438.
70. Koren, S., Fleischmann, W.R., Circadian variations in myelosuppressive activity of interferon-α in mice: identification of an optimal treatment time associated with reduced myelosuppressive activity. *Exp. Hematol.* 1993; 21:552–559.
71. Koren, S., Fleischmann, W.R., Optimal circadian timing reduces the myelosuppressive activity of rMuIFN-γ administered to mice. *J. Interferon Res.* 1993; 13:187–194.
72. Abrams, P.G., McClamrock, E., Foon, K.A., Evening administration of alpha interferon. *N. Engl. J. Med.* 1985; 312:443–444 (Letter to the editor).
73. Brummer, P.D., Levi, F., DiPalma, M. et al., A phase I trial of 21-day continuous venous infusion of α-interferon at circadian rhythm modulated rate in cancer patients. *J. Immunol.* 1991; 10:440–447.
74. Smith, D., Wagstaff, J., Thatcher, N., Scarffe, H., A phase-I study of rDNA alpha-2b interferon as a 6 week continuous intravenous infusion. *Cancer Chemother. Pharmacol.* 1987; 20:327–331.

75. Muss, H.B., Costanzi, J.J., Leavitt, R. et al., Recombinant alpha interferon in renal cell carcinoma: a randomized trial of two routes of administration. *J. Clin. Oncol.* 1987; 5:286–291.

76. Koren, S., Whorton, E.J., Fleischmann, W.J., Circadian dependence of interferon antitumor activity in mice. *J. Natl. Cancer Inst.* 1993; 85:1927–1932.

77. English, J., Aherne, G.W., Marks, V., The effect of timing of a single injection on the toxicity of methotrexate in the rat. *Cancer Chemother. Pharmacol.* 1982; 9:114–117.

78. Kodama, M., Kodama, T., Influence of corticosteroid hormones on the therapeutic efficacy of cyclophosphamide. *Gann* 1982; 73:661–666.

79. Shepherd, R., Harrap, K.R., Modulation of the toxicity and antitumor activity of alkylating drugs by steroids. *Br. J. Cancer* 1982; 45:413.

80. Lévi, F., Halberg, F., Haus, E. et al., Synthetic adrenocorticotropin for optimizing murine circadian chronotolerance for adriamycin. *Chronobiologia* 1980; 7:227–244.

81. Rivard, G., Infante-Rivard, C., Hoyoux, C., Champagne, J., Maintenance chemotherapy for childhood acute lymphoblastic leukemia: better in the evening. *Lancet* 1985; 2:1264–1266.

82. Petrie, K., Dawson, A.G., Thompson, L., Brook, R., A double blind trial of melatonin as a treatment for jet lag in international cabin crew. *Biol-Psychiatry* 1993; 33:526–530.

83. Carter, D.S., Goldman, B.D., Antigonadal effects of timed melatonin infusion in pinealectomised male Djungarian hamsters (*Phodopus sungorus sungorus*): duration is the critical parameter. *Endocrinology* 1983; 113:1267–1267.

84. Manning, M.C., Patel, K., Borchardt, R.T., Stability of protein pharmaceuticals. *Pharm. Res.* 1989; 6:903.

85. Trissel, L.A., *Handbook of Injectable Drugs*. Bethesda: American Society of Hospital Pharmacists, 1990:261, 422, 456, 564.

86. Andrade, J.D., Hlady, V., Protein adsorption and materials compatibility: a tutorial review and suggested hypothesis. *Adv. Polym. Sci.* 1986; 79:1.

87. Gu, L.C., Erdos, E.A., Chiang, H.S. et al., Stability of interleukin 1β (IL-1β) in aqueous solution: analytical methods, kinetics, products and solution formulation implications. *Pharm. Res.* 1991; 8:245.

88. Florence, A.T., *Drug Delivery Systems of the Future*. Vol. 4. Greenford, Middlesex, U.K.: Duncan, Flockhard, 1988.

89. Geigert, J., Overview of the stability and handling of recombinant protein drugs. *J. Parenter. Sci. Technol.* 1989; 43:220.

90. Tzannis, S.T., Pryzbycien, T.M., Hrushesky, W.J.M., Wood, P., The impact of formulated interleukin-2/delivery device surface interactions on bioefficacy. *Materials Research Soc. Symp. Proc.* 1994; 331:227–232.

91. Theeuwes, F., Yum, S.I., Haak, R., Wong, P., Systems for triggered, pulsed and programmed drug delivery, *Temporal Control of Drug Delivery*, New York, 1991. Vol. 618. *Ann. N.Y. Acad. Sci.*

92. Lanning, R.M., Hrushesky, W.J.M., Outpatient time-specified infusion of fluoropyrimidines by implanted pump is less costly than flat delivery by external pump. *Prog. Clin. Biol. Res.* 1990; 341B:397–409.

93. Korsmeyer, R.W., Diffusion controlled systems: hydrogels. In Tarcha, P.J., Ed. *Polymers for Controlled Drug Delivery*. Boca Raton, FL: CRC Press, 1991:15–37.

94. Borodkin, S., Ion-exchange resin delivery systems. In Tarcha, P.J., Ed. *Polymers for Controlled Drug Delivery*. Boca Raton, FL: CRC Press, 1991:215–230.

95. Pecosky, D.A., Robinson, J.R., Bioadhesive polymers and drug delivery. In Tarcha, P.J., Ed. *Polymers for Controlled Drug Delivery*. Boca Raton, FL: CRC Press, 1991:99–125.

96. Ranney, D.F., Huffaker, H.H., Magnetic microspheres for the targeted controlled release of drugs and diagnostic agents. In: *Ann. N.Y. Acad. Sci., Biological Approaches to the Controlled Delivery of Drugs,* 1987. Vol. 507.

Section II
Fundamentals

3 Electrical Properties of Skin

Jagdish Singh, Steven M. Dinh, and Bret Berner

CONTENTS

3.1 INTRODUCTION

Electrically enhanced drug delivery through skin has recently received increased attention as a means for systemic delivery of ionized drugs.[1-4] Although there has been an awareness of ionic transport through human skin for many years,[5-7] the scientific focus has been nonpolar transport through skin.[8] With the exception of the classic work of Rosendahl,[9-11] the review by Tregear,[5] and extensive interest in relating transepidermal water loss to impedance by the cosmetic industry,[12-14] the electrochemistry of skin has only recently received attention. In particular, the feasibility of iontophoresis is being assessed *in vitro* and *in vivo*[15-18] with increasing use of classic electrochemical techniques.[19]

One quickly finds in the laboratory that, while it is possible to increase the skin penetration rates of many ionic compounds using iontophoresis, the efficiency with which this is accomplished is often not very high. Much of the electric current is

0-8493-7681-5/98/$0.00+$.50
© 1998 by CRC Press LLC

carried by ions other than the drug ion of interest. In particular, the presence of substantial concentrations of sodium and chloride ions in the skin inevitably leads to a situation in which the drug ion competes as the charge carrier with one or the other of these small, relatively mobile ions.[20] Since the total amount of current that can be passed through the skin is limited by the battery of the iontophoretic device and by the tolerance of the patient to the treatment, the efficiency of iontophoretic delivery becomes a key question in determining its practical value for a particular drug therapy. In order to predict the efficiency of iontophoretic delivery, one must first understand electrical properties of the skin. This chapter deals with the electrical properties of the skin *in vitro* and *in vivo*.

3.2 PRINCIPLES

3.2.1 PARAMETERS

If a system is unchanged by the passage of current and does not itself supply energy to the current, then the current through it is proportional to the electromotive force (e.m.f.) across it (Ohm's law). This is exactly analogous to Fick's law of diffusion. For a direct current (DC):

$$V = iR_0 \tag{3.1}$$

where V = voltage, i = current, R_0 = resistance.

For a sinusoidally oscillating current (AC) of frequency f:

$$V_m = i_m Z_f \tag{3.2}$$

where V_m and i_m are the time averages (root mean square) of the voltage and current. Z_f is termed the impedance at frequency f.

During the passage of an alternating current, charge accumulates in different parts of the system if there are thin, highly resistive membranes within it, i.e., a capacitance. As a result of this capacitance, the current precedes the voltage; i.e., the current maximum will be reached earlier than the voltage maximum. This difference is specified by the phase angle (ϕ); if $\phi = 0°$ the voltage and current rise and fall together. If it is 90°, the current maximum occurs as the voltage is zero. The two parameters, Z and ϕ, completely define the response of an ohmic system to AC. The system may also be specified in a different, but parallel manner. Supposing that during the passage of AC of frequency f, the voltage across the system is V_1 when the current is at its maximum and V_0 when the current is zero, we define two proportionality constants, R_f and X_f, such that

$$V_1 = i_m R_f$$

$$V_0 = i_m X_f$$

X_f is termed reactance, R_f the resistance, at frequency f.

The root mean square value of the e.m.f., V_m, can be shown to be

$$V_m = \sqrt{V_1^2 + V_0^2}$$

$$V_m = \sqrt{R_f^2 + X_f^2}$$

$$Z_f = \sqrt{R_f^2 + X_f^2} \tag{3.3}$$

and also

$$\tan \phi = \frac{X_f}{R_f} \tag{3.4}$$

Hence the ohmic behavior at frequency f can be completely specified either by X_f, R_f, or by Z, ϕ. Note that X_f and R_f may vary with the frequency f. The response to DC is simply a special case of Equations 3.3 and 3.4: at $f = 0$, $R_f = R_0$ and $\tan \phi_0 = 0$, $Z_0 = R_0$. The application of these parameters depends upon the validity of Ohm's law, just as the use of a permeability constant depends on Fick's law. Both laws indicate that the system remains passive and is unaffected.

3.2.1.1   The Ohmic Electrical Properties of Skin

Fricke[21] produced the following theory of electrolytic polarization, i.e., the behavior of a metal carrying a current immersed in an electrolyte solution. The passage of a charge across the system produces a back e.m.f. (V) which decays as some power (m) of time after the charge has passed.

$$V = V_o t^{-m} \quad (0 < m < 1) \tag{3.5}$$

Hence, the impedance across the system may be related to the frequency of the applied AC, and the phase angle is constant:

$$\phi = (1 - m) \frac{\pi}{2} \tag{3.6}$$

and the impedance is inversely related to a power of the frequency[22]:

$$Z = k f^{m-1} \tag{3.7}$$

Any system in which passage of a current produces a back voltage that decays as a power function of time with an exponent less than unity obeys Equations 3.6 and

3.7. Such a system is called a "polarization impedance" after the initial physical example, but the occurrence of such an impedance does not imply any chemical reactions within the system. For instance, when a current passes into a system composed of a lot of resistors and capacitors connected in series and parallel, a voltage is created across the system which decays according to the various time constants of the elements of the system. If there are many elements in the system, the decay may approximate the power law of Equation 3.5. In that case the system will behave as a polarization impedance, even though no chemical changes have occurred. Cellular tissues often behave as polarization impedances,[23] because cell membranes behave as tiny capacitors, and the intercellular channels as shunt resistance pathways. When cells are free in suspension, the electrical capacity of their cell membranes may be deduced from their polarization impedance.[24]

3.3   ELECTRICAL PROPERTIES OF EXCISED SKIN

3.3.1   IMPEDANCE SPECTROSCOPY

Impedance spectroscopy is the measurement of the conductive and capacitative properties of electrically active systems over a broad range of frequencies. It has been applied extensively to the investigation of transport in biological membranes[21-23] and in battery and sensor research.[25]

   In impedance spectroscopy, a small sinusoidal perturbation in potential V at a fixed frequency, ω, is applied to the system and the current response is measured. This current response I, does not only vary in magnitude, but is shifted by a phase angle ϕ. The entire frequency spectrum is measured and data may be handled conveniently as a Bode plot, that is, $\log |Z|$ versus $\log \omega$ where Z is the complete impedance. For a simple resistor, the impedance is a constant and a Bode plot for this resistor is a horizontal line. A capacitor would produce a line with a slope of -1; that is, for a capacitor:

$$Z = i/\omega C \qquad (3.8)$$

   In his classic studies of the impedance of skin, Rosendahl[9-11] modeled the *in vitro* electrical properties of skin at low voltages as a parallel resistor and capacitor. To fit the data accurately, a resistor in series should be added to account for the properties of the solution.[26] This equivalent circuit and a theoretical fit of its electrical behavior to the measured impedance of the skin are shown in Figure 3.1. For low voltages, this sample circuit is clearly adequate to describe the electrical properties of skin. The zero frequency asymptote is the sum of the two resistances, and the high frequency asymptote is the resistance of solution. The roll-off reflects the RC circuit. While the capacitance of skin is relatively reproducible, the resistance of skin is highly variable from 5 to 100 kΩ/cm^2.[26]

   As typifies the impedance of biological membranes and polymers, the capacitative properties of the membrane are nonideal and optimal curve fitting may be obtained by treating these properties as $Z_c = Ke^{\alpha C}$,[3] where α may vary between 0 and 1 and is typically 0.8 for stratum corneum (SC).[5]

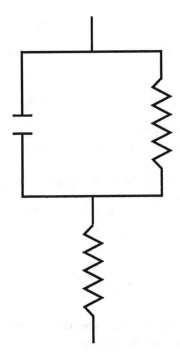

FIGURE 3.1 An equivalent circuit for skin.

3.3.2 CHARACTERIZATION OF EXCISED SKIN

Impedance spectroscopy, constant current iontophoresis, and potentiometry have been used to characterize ionic transport through human epidermis *in vitro* by DeNuzzio and Berner.[26] A resistor (solution resistance) in series with a parallel combination of resistance and capacitance (membrane) is an equivalent circuit for epidermis. Impedance is used to investigate the electrical response of skin to different ions, applied currents, and fields. The flux–current relationships for a solute through human skin are characterized *in vitro*, and the reversibility of iontophoresis is monitored by simultaneous impedance spectroscopy. Potentiometry permits the study of the selectivity of the skin to different ions. The proportion of current carried by an ion in an electrolyte is known as the transport number of the ion (t_i). The transport numbers of various ions in human skin were determined from potentiometric measurements. Potentiometry is the measurement of the potential of a system at zero net current.[27] For an electrochemical cell comprising a membrane (epidermis) separating different concentrations of an electrolyte and silver–silver chloride electrodes:

$$Ag, AgCl \, |[electrolyte1]| \, epidermis \, |[electrolyte2]| \, Ag, AgCl \qquad (3.9)$$

The total potential of the system comprises the sum of the potential difference of the electrodes and the membrane potential.

$$E_{system} = \Delta E_{electrodes} + E_{membrane} \tag{3.10}$$

The potential difference due to Ag, AgCl electrodes can be calculated from the Nernst equation:

$$\Delta E_{electrodes} = RT/F \ln (\alpha_1/\alpha_2) \tag{3.11}$$

where R is the gas constant, T is the absolute temperature, and F is Faraday's constant (96485 C/eq). The activities of solutions 1 and 2 (α_1 and α_2) are approximated by the respective concentrations in dilute solutions.

The activity gradient across the membrane gives rise to a membrane potential. As ions diffuse at different rates, a potential develops due to charge separation. By assuming that transport numbers are independent of concentration, the membrane potential is related to the transport numbers of the ions in the system by

$$E_{membranes} = \frac{RT}{F} \sum \int_1^2 \frac{t_i}{z_i} d(\ln \alpha_i) \tag{3.12}$$

where z_i is the valence of the ion. For a standard concentration cell with the same salt on both sides of the membrane, this equation reduces to

$$E_{membranes} = \frac{-RT}{F} \left[\frac{t_+}{z_+} \ln \frac{a_{+2}}{a_{+1}} + \frac{t_-}{z_-} \ln \frac{a_{-2}}{a_{-1}} \right] \tag{3.13}$$

Assuming that all of the current is carried by ions yields $t_+ + t_- = 1$. By using the dilute solution approximation for the mean ionic activity, concentrations (c_i) may be substituted for activities. Therefore, for a simple 1:1 electrolyte (e.g., KCl), $z_+ = -z_- = 1$, the membrane potential is given by

$$E_{membranes} = \frac{-RT}{F}(2t_+ - 1)\ln \frac{[c_2]}{[c_1]} \tag{3.14}$$

For a 2:1 electrolyte such as $CaCl_2$, the membrane potential is given by

$$E_{membranes} = \frac{-RT}{F}\left(\frac{3t_+}{2-1}\right)\ln \frac{[c_2]}{[c_1]} \tag{3.15}$$

The ion selectivity of human epidermis can be determined by measuring the potential difference generated by an epidermal membrane separating two chloride salt solutions of different concentrations.[26] Within the alkali metals, human epidermis is cation selective, but not size selective.

While iontophoretic transport appears to obey simple laws for transport through a restricted aqueous volume fraction with some slight degree of cation selectivity, the transport of divalent ions and the long relaxation of the impedance after iontophoresis suggest nonlinear phenomena. A description of these behaviors and two interpretations will be presented in a later section. Oh et al.[28] studied the effect of current, ionic strength, and temperature on the electrical properties of hairless mouse skin. The complex electrical impedance of hairless mouse skin was measured as a function of frequency, and the resistance and capacitance were determined. Increasing the ionic strength of the bathing medium and increasing the magnitude of current decreased resistance, whereas capacitance was, in general, unchanged. These changes occurred rapidly. The decrease in resistance with increasing the ionic strength of the bathing medium was consistent with elevated ion levels within the ion-conducting pathways of the membrane. The decrease in resistance by increasing the magnitude of current seems to be related to alteration of the current-conducting pathway. With increasing temperature, resistance also decreased while capacitance increased. The activation energy for ion conduction through the skin was estimated to be 3.4 kcal/mol at physiologically relevant temperatures. The most-marked changes occurred at the phase transition temperature (60°C) of the SC lipids where the resistance decreased precipitously and the capacitance steadily increased. Ultimately, the impedance became independent of frequency, suggesting that the capacitative properties of the barrier had been lost. Overall, the results provide mechanistic insight into ion conduction through the skin and into the role of SC lipids in skin capacitance. Thus, impedance spectroscopy of skin is a powerful tool with which to probe the electrical properties of the skin, and to examine how perturbation of a membrane (by temperature, iontophoresis, ionic strength, and penetration enhancer treatment) can be analyzed.[26] Furthermore, temperature- and ionic strength–dependent changes in R suggest that conduction through the SC is primarily associated with an aqueous pathway distinct from the intercellular lipid domains, which comprise the main contribution to the skin capacitance.

3.3.3 NONLINEAR ELECTRICAL PROPERTIES OF SKIN

Rosendahl[9,10] described the decline in the resistance of skin at constant current. Numerous investigators commented on this decline of the resistance of skin with time during iontophoresis.[26,29-31] The electrical resistance of skin is bound by an upper limit at equilibrium and a lower limit at steady state (Figure 3.2).[32] This lower limit of the steady-state resistance of skin substantially reduces the power or battery requirements for iontophoresis.

These nonlinear properties of skin may be quantitatively interpreted in terms of a model of negatively charged pores.[32] A master curve may be constructed for this steady-state resistance in which $\log (R_{\text{skin resistance}}/R_{\text{solution resistance}})$ is plotted (Figure 3.3) vs. $\log (I \text{ current density/salt concentration } C_0)$. In this manner the varying effects of current density and salt concentration can be interpreted. The slope observed in Figure 3.3 is -0.65. For a cylindrical pore, conductive and convective transport were modeled, and a cubic equation in R/R_{solution} was obtained. In the limit of pure conduction,

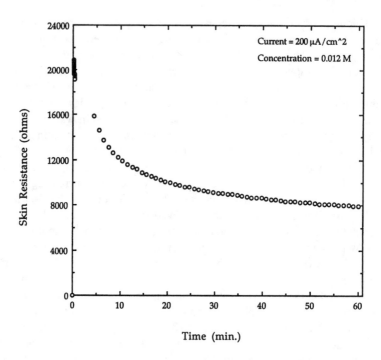

FIGURE 3.2   Transient behavior of skin electrical resistance during iontophoresis.

$$\left(R/R_{\text{solution}}\right) \propto \left(I/C_0\right)^0 \tag{3.16}$$

That is, for conductive transport, at small current densities ohmic behavior is observed. For pure convection through charged pores, as has been suggested by Pikal[38] to occur in iontophoresis, one predicts that

$$\left(R/R_{\text{solution}}\right) \propto \left(I/C_0\right)^{-2/3} \tag{3.17}$$

Given the agreement between the theoretical slope of –2/3 and the experimental data, convective transport would appear to dominate at the practical current densities used in iontophoresis.

The equilibrium resistance, i.e., the resistance at long times at zero current, is quite sensitive to the pore geometry and it may be shown that:

$$\left(R/R_{\text{solution}}\right)_{\text{equilibrium}} \propto \left(\sigma L_{\text{sc}}/\upsilon L_{\text{soln}}\right) \tag{3.18}$$

where σ is the tortuosity, L_{sc} is the thickness of the SC, and υ is the porosity. For the equilibrium resistance, the estimated pore radius, surface charge, and the ratio

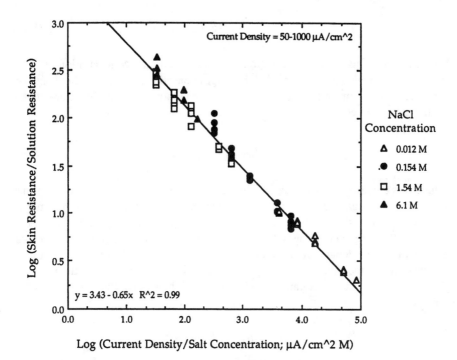

FIGURE 3.3   Master curve of the steady-state electrical resistance of skin.

of porosity to tortuosity are 0.25 nm, -0.05 C/m^2, and 10^{-7}, respectively. The pore radius has been estimated to be 0.18, 0.18, and 0.3 nm by Inamori et al.,[33] Ruddy and Hadzija,[34] and Yoshida and Roberts,[35] respectively. The effective porosity is considerably less than the area fraction of hair follicles and sweat glands of 10^{-4} to 10^{-3}.

An alternative model has been proposed by Scott et al.[36] where the number of pores or area fraction of pores varies with current density. Creation of pores in a lipid bilayer requires on the order of 1 V,[37] and to create pores in the SC on the order of 50 bilayers in series would require some 50 V to create such pores in skin. A similar result would be obtained using the elasticity of skin in a calculation. This is in general agreement with the data on electroporation through skin. At these large applied voltages, enormous rapid decreases in the resistance of skin have been observed, and the time scale for recovery of this resistance is on the order of minutes. These changes have been modeled in terms of creation of straight-through pores.

3.3.4   IONTOPHORETIC TRANSPORT THROUGH SKIN

3.3.4.1   Diffusive Regime

At low current densities or small voltages, diffusive transport is the dominant mechanism of ion transport through skin. Electrodiffusion of an ideal species i in the absence of convection is governed by the Nernst–Planck[20] equation:

$$J_i = -D_i\left(dC_i/dx\right) - \left(D_i z_i FC_i/RT\right)\left(dV/dx\right) \tag{3.19}$$

where J is the flux, D is the diffusion coefficient, C is the concentration, z is the charge, V is the electrical potential, R is the gas constant, F is the Faraday constant, T is the absolute temperature, and x is the distance within the membrane. Consistency with the Poisson equation[32] is also required, and

$$\left(d^2V/dx^2\right) = -\left(\rho/\varepsilon\right) \tag{3.20}$$

where ρ is the charge density and ε is the electric permittivity. While other regimes have been investigated with respect to iontophoretic transport, the most informative treatment is the constant field or Goldman approximation[20] in which the Debye length or the characteristic length of the surface charge layer is much greater than the characteristic length of the membrane. Under this approximation, the iontophoretic flux at the dimensionless potential, υ, where $\upsilon = zF\Delta V/RT$ is the potential difference across the membrane, may be related to the passive flux at $v = 0$, by the equation:

$$J(v)/J(0) = v\big/\left(1 - e^{-v}\right) \tag{3.21}$$

Kasting and Bowman[44] observed that the limit of validity of Equation 3.9 was 0.25 V for the iontophoretic transport of disodium etidronate, a multiply charged anionic bisphosphonate. Fluxes greater than theory were observed at high voltages, and convective transport should be included in the theoretical model. Particularly, changes in the resistance of skin at the previously discussed higher current densities or voltages were observed.

The time lag to obtain the steady-state flux, t_L, was found to be[20]

$$t_L(v)/t_L(0) = \left(6/\upsilon^2\right)\left(\upsilon\coth(\upsilon/2) - 2\right) \tag{3.22}$$

However, the experimental decrease in the time lag was not as large as predicted.

3.3.4.2 Convective Flow and Electro-Osmosis

The most complete treatment of electro-osmotic flow through skin was presented in the series of articles by Pikal and Shah,[38,39] and a summary of the predictions are presented here.

The SC is treated as a collection of three sets of identical pores: positively charged, neutral, and negatively charged. These respective radii for these pores are 9, 18, and 36 Å.[38]

The total iontophoretic or electroosmotic flux is the sum of the fluxes through each set of pores and may be modeled as

$$J(\upsilon)/j(0) = \Sigma A_j \alpha_j \left(1 - \exp\left(-\alpha_j\right)\right) \tag{3.23}$$

where A_j is the area fraction of each type of pore and α_j is a flux enhancement parameter. In a thorough theoretical treatment based on Mannings model, Pikal and Shah[39] express α in terms of υ, the pore radius, the Debye length, and the surface charge density. This model is consistent with the observation of both cathodal and anodal electro-osmosis of mannitol through skin.[40] Anions, especially cations, and neutral species all show large flux enhancements.

3.3.5 THE ROUTE OF IONTOPHORETIC TRANSPORT

It has been proposed that ion transport may also occur through highly conductive pathways, not associated with the skin appendages.[4,36] Since appendages and other highly conductive pathways make up a very small percentage of the total skin surface,[41] nonappendageal ion transport (involving the SC lipids lamellar matrix) may also contribute substantially to the net flux through skin under both passive and iontophoretic conditions. If the SC lipid route contributes to ion transport, then the accessibility of the lamellae interior to these charged species should increase. Recently, oleic acid was found to increase the passive and iontophoretic transdermal transport of ionic solute (luteinizing hormone–releasing hormone) by increasing the SC lipid fluidity.[17] Pechtold et al.[42] studied the influence of an electric field on ion and water accessibility to SC lipid lamellae. The results show that in the presence of an applied electric field the SC lipid lamellae interior becomes more accessible to water and ions. These results imply that during iontophoresis, ion and water transport through human skin is associated, at least in part, with the SC lipid lamellae. More-detailed mechanistic studies may provide the investigator with a means to optimize electrically enhanced, transdermal drug delivery systems.

3.4 ELECTRICAL PROPERTIES OF FROZEN EXCISED SKIN

While the use of human cadaver skin *in vitro* for studying the passive diffusion of drugs across skin is firmly established,[5] less is known about the utility of this technique for studying iontophoretic drug delivery. The use of skin that has been stored frozen poses the additional question of tissue integrity. Frozen, excised human skin obtained from skin banks has received widespread use in skin penetration studies. Franz[43] and others have shown that such tissue can give drug permeation rates which are comparable to those obtained with fresh skin *in vitro* and to the results of human *in vivo* studies. Less is known about the utility of this tissue for studying the permeation of ions. Since ionic penetration rates through skin are extremely low, it seemed possible that defects induced by the freezing process might grossly alter the permeability of the tissue to ions, rendering it useless for such studies. DeNuzzio and Berner in a series of unpublished experiments demonstrated that isolated epidermis stored frozen retained its ion selectivity for only 1 month.

Kasting and Bowman[44] studied the DC current–voltage relationships and sodium ion transport measurements for human allograft skin immersed in saline buffers using a four-terminal potentiometric method and diffusion cells. About three fourths of the skin samples were deemed suitable for study on the basis of their high resistivities and similar flux–voltage characteristics. Most of these samples yielded sodium ion permeability coefficients less than or equal to those reported for human skin *in vivo*. The current–voltage relationship in these tissues was time dependent, highly nonlinear, and slightly asymmetric with respect to the sign of the applied potential. Skin resistance decreased as current or voltage increased. For current densities less than 15 $\mu A/cm^2$ and exposure times of 10 to 20 min, this decrease was almost completely reversible; at higher current densities, both reversible and irreversible effects were observed. The overall dependence of current on voltage was nearly exponential. Diffusion potentials, sodium ion membrane transference numbers, and sodium ion flux enhancement factors during iontophoresis were measured for skin immersed both in normal saline solutions and in saline solutions of differing concentrations. The sign of the diffusion potentials and the value of the sodium ion transference number (0.51 in normal saline at pH 7.4) indicated a weak permselectivity of the skin for transport of sodium ion vs. chloride. At a current density of 71 $\mu A/cm^2$ and transmembrane potentials in the range of 1.1 to 1.6 V, the flux enhancement for sodium ion was three to five times greater than that predicted for an uncharged homogeneous membrane according to electrodiffusion theory. For transmembrane potentials less than 0.17 V, agreement of this theory with the data was better but still incomplete.

In conclusion, frozen, excised human skin has been shown to be a promising tissue for conducting iontophoresis studies, provided the tissue is properly prepared and electrically prescreened for defects. Ionic transport in this tissue cannot be adequately predicted by theories involving an uncharged, homogeneous membrane with equilibrium boundary conditions. A theory incorporating kinetic barriers to charge transport or, as previously discussed, negatively charged pores may better explain the observed phenomena.

3.5   ELECTRICAL PROPERTIES OF SKIN *IN VIVO*

The basic parallel RC-circuit model for a biological membrane has an impedance given by

$$Z_m = \frac{R_m}{1 + j\omega C_m R_m} \qquad (3.24)$$

where Z_m = membrane impedance, R_m = membrane resistance, C_m = membrane capacitance, and ω = angular frequency (rad s^{-1}).

A more accurate representation replaces the capacitor with a constant-phase element (CPE). A CPE can be considered as having a phase-angle of $\alpha\pi/2$, where α is a frequency-independent constant that determines the distance below the real-axis of the center of the impedance locus. It has an impedance of the form, $I/A(j\omega)^{\alpha}$, where A is a constant. When $\alpha = 1$, the CPE behaves as an ideal capacitor; when

$\alpha = 0$, it behaves as a pure resistor. The impedance of a parallel R-CPE circuit is given by

$$Z_m = \frac{R_m}{1+(j\omega)^\alpha AR_m} \tag{3.25}$$

The center of the locus in the complex plane impedance plot for a parallel R-CPE circuit is characteristically depressed, as observed for skin.

Kalia and Guy[45] investigated the electrical charateristics of human skin *in vivo*. Passage of an iontophoretic current caused a significant reduction in the magnitude of the skin impedance. Increasing the current density caused an even greater reduction in the value of the skin impedance and slowed the rate of recovery. Reduction of the ionic strength resulted in an increase in the rate of recovery following iontophoresis. A significant increase in the rate of recovery was observed when $CaCl_2$ replaced NaCl as the electrolyte. Although visual inspection revealed the presence of greater erythema when $CaCl_2$ was used, there was an absence of the mild sensation experienced by volunteers when using NaCl. The data were fitted to an equivalent circuit consisting of a resistor in parallel with constant-phase element and a mechanistic model proposed to explain the electrical properties of the skin. This is a comprehensive investigation of the effect of iontophoresis on the electrical properties of human skin *in vivo*. It would appear from the results, and from their interpretation, that impedance spectroscopy may be an effective method to quantify the impact of iontophoresis on the skin, and to determine the extent to which proposed drug delivery regimens will perturb skin barrier function.

3.6   CONCLUSION

The basic work on the electrical properties of skin has been investigated. The subject is closely akin to the study of skin permeability; electrical measurements are a simple means of testing the permeability of skin to the ions within the SC. Impedance spectroscopy of the skin is a powerful tool to probe the electrical properties of the skin. Measurement of the impedance of the skin may provide a noninvasive quantifiable method to determine the tissue-altering properties of electrical currents. Clear insight into the mechanism of iontophoresis is obtained by a combination of models of diffusion–convection through pores and electrochemical studies. Impedance spectroscopy may also be an effective method to quantify the impact of iontophoresis on the skin barrier.

REFERENCES

1. A. Banga and Y.W. Chien, Iontophoretic delivery of drugs: fundamentals, developments, and biomedical applications, *J. Controlled Release,* 7: 1–24 (1988).
2. R.R. Burnette and D. Marrero, Comparison between the iontophoretic and passive transport of thyrotropin releasing hormone across excised nude mouse skin, *J. Pharm. Sci.,* 75: 738–743 (1986).

3. B.R. Meyer, W. Kreis, J. Eshbach, V. O'Mara, S. Rosen, and D. Sibalis, Successful transdermal administration of therapeutic doses of a polypeptide to normal human volunteers, *Clin. Pharmacol. Ther.*, 44: 607–612 (1988).

4. J. Singh and K.S. Bhatia, Topical iontophoretic drug delivery: pathway, principles, factors, and skin irritation, *Med. Res. Rev.*, 16: 285–29 (1996).

5. R.T. Tregear, *Physical Functions of Skin*, Academic Press, London, pp. 53–72 (1966).

6. H. Molitor and L. Fernandez, Studies on iontophoresis, *Am. J. Med. Sci.*, 198: 778–785 (1939).

7. H.A. Abramson and M.H. Gorin, Skin reactions IX. The electrophoretic demonstration of the patent pores of the living human skin, its relation to the change of skin, *J. Phys. Chem.*, 44: 1094–1102 (1940).

8. R.J. Scheuplein and I.H. Blank, Permeability of the skin, *Physiol. Rev.*, 51: 702–747 (1971).

9. T. Rosendahl, Studies on the conducting properties of human skin to direct current, *Acta Physiol. Scand.*, 5: 130–151 (1943).

10. T. Rosendahl, Further studies on the conducting properties of human skin to direct and alternating current, *Acta Physiol. Scand.*, 8: 183–202 (1944).

11. T. Rosendahl, Concluding studies on the conducting properties of human skin to alternating current, *Acta Physiol. Scand.*, 9: 39–49 (1945).

12. Y. Yamamoto and T. Yamamoto, Measurement of electrical bioimpedance and its applications, *Med. Prog. Technol.*, 12: 171–183 (1987).

13. T. Yamamoto and Y. Yamamoto, Electrical properties of epidermal stratum corneum, *Med. Biol. Eng.*, 14: 151–158 (1976).

14. T. Yamamoto and Y. Yamamoto, Analysis for the change of skin impedance, *Med. Biol. Eng. Comput.*, 15: 219–227 (1977).

15. J. Singh and M.S. Roberts, Iontophoretic transport of amphoteric solutes through human epidermis: P-aminobenzoic acid and amphotericin, *Pharm. Sci.*, 1: 223–226 (1995).

16. J. Singh, M. Gross, M. O'Connell, B. Sage, and H.I. Maibach, Effect of iontophoresis in different ethnic groups' skin function, *Int. Symp. Control. Rel. Bioact. Mater.*, 21: 365–366 (1994).

17. K.S. Bhatia and J. Singh, Effect of penetration enhancer and iontophoresis on the LHRH permeability and FT-IR spectroscopy, *Int. Symp. Control. Rel. Bioact. Mater.*, 23: 287–288 (1996).

18. S. Ganga, P.R. Rao, and J. Singh, Transdermal delivery of metoprolol *in vivo* by iontophoresis and passive diffusion from matrix controlled transdermal patches, *Pharm. Res.*, 10: S 225 (1993).

19. R.R. Burnette and B. Ongipipattanakal, Characterization of the pore transport properties and tissue alteration of excised human skin during iontophoresis, *J. Pharm. Sci.*, 77: 132–137 (1988).

20. G.B. Kasting and J.C. Keister, Application of electrodiffusion theory for a homogeneous membrane to iontophoretic transport through skin, *J. Controlled Release*, 8: 195–210 (1989).

21. H. Fricke, The theory of electrolytic polarization. *Philos. Mag.* 14: 310–318 (1932).

22. A. Barnett, The phase angle of normal human skin, *J. Physiol.*, 93: 349–366 (1938).

23. K.S. Cole, Electric phase angle of cell membrane, *J. Gen. Physiol.* 15: 641–649 (1932).

24. H. Pauly, Electrical properties of cytoplasmic membrane and the cytoplasm of bacteria and protoplasts, *Bio-Med. Electron.*, 9: 93–95 (1962).

25. D.D. Macdonald, *Transient Techniques in Electrochemistry*, Plenum Press, New York (1977).

26. J.D. DeNuzzio and B. Berner, Electrochemical and iontophoretic studies of human skin, *J. Controlled. Release,* 11: 105–112 (1990).

27. F. Helfferich, *Ion Exchange,* McGraw-Hill, New York, pp. 371–378 (1962).

28. S.Y. Oh, L. Leung, D. Bommannan, R.H. Guy, and R.O. Potts, Effect of current, ionic strength and temperature on the electrical properties of skin, *J. Controlled Release,* 27: 115–125 (1993).

29. R. Edelberg, T. Greiner, and N.R. Burch, Some membrane properties in the galvanic skin response, *Arch. Neurol. Psychiat.,* 7: 163–169 (1960).

30. A.C. Cleves and J.F. Sumner, The measurement of human capacitance and resistance in relation to electrostatic hazards with primary explosives, *Explos. Res. Dev. Establ. Rep.,* 18: R.62 (1962)

31. R.R. Burnette and T.M. Bagniefski, Influence of constant current iontophoresis on the impedance and passive Na^+ permeability of excised nude mouse skin, *J. Pharm. Sci.,* 77: 492–497 (1988).

32. S. M. Dinh, C.W. Luo, and B. Berner, Upper and lower limits of human skin electrical resistance in iontophoresis. *AIChE J.,* 39: 2011–2018 (1993).

33. T. Inamori, A.H. Ghanem, and W.I. Higuchi, Estimation of pore size of ethanol pretreated human epidermal membrane using polystyrene sulfonate, *Proc. Int. Symp. Control. Rel. Bioact. Mater.,* 19:474 (1992).

34. S.B. Ruddy and B.A. Hadzija, Iontophoretic permeability of polyethylene glycols through hairless rat skin: application of hydrodynamic theory for hindered transport through liquid-filled pores, *Drug Dev. Discovery,* 8:207 (1992).

35. N.H. Yoshida and M.S. Roberts, Structure-transport relationships in transdermal iontophoresis, *Adv. Drug Delivery Rev.,* 9,239 (1992).

36. E.R. Scott, A.I. Laplaza, H.S. White, and J.B. Phipps, Transport of ionic species in skin: contribution of pores to the overall skin conductance, *Pharm. Res.,* 10: 1699–1709 (1993).

37. Y.A. Chizmadzhev, V.G. Zarnitsin, J.C. Weaver, and R. O. Potts, Mechanism of electroinduced ionic species transport through a multilamellar lipid system, *Biophys. J.* 68: 749–765 (1995).

38. M.J. Pikal, The role of electroosmotic flow in transdermal iontophoresis, *Adv. Drug Delivery Rev.,* 9:201–237 (1992).

39. M.J. Pikal and S. Shah, Transport mechanisms in iontophoresis III: an experimental study of the contributions of electroosmotic flow and permeability change in transport of low and high molecular weight solutes, *Pharm. Res.,* 7, 222–229 (1990).

40. A. Kim, P.G. Green, G. Rao, and R.H. Guy, Convective solvent flow across the skin during iontophoresis, *Pharm. Res.,* 10:1315–1320 (1993).

41. H. Schaeffer, F. Watts, J. Brod, and B. Illel, Follicular penetration. In R.C. Scott, R.H. Guy, and J. Hadgraft, Eds., *Prediction of Percutaneous Penetration: Methods, Measurements, and Modeling,* IBC Technical Services, London, pp. 163–173 (1990).

42. L.A.R.M. Pechtold, W. Abraham, and R.O. Potts, The influence of an electric field on ion and water accessibility to stratum corneum lipid lamellae, *Pharm. Res.,* 13: 1168–1173 (1996).

43. T.J. Franz, Percutaneous absorption. On the relevance of *in vitro* data, *J. Invest. Dermatol.,* 64: 190–195 (1975).

44. G.B. Kasting and L.A. Bowman, DC electrical properties of frozen, excised human skin, *Pharm. Res.,* 7: 134–143 (1990).

45. Y.N. Kalia and R.H. Guy, The electrical characteristics of human skin *in vivo, Pharm. Res.,* 12: 1605–1613 (1995).

4 Skin Tolerability: Irritation*

Smita Amin and Howard I. Maibach

CONTENTS

---

* Adapted from Weltfriend et al.[1]

0-8493-7681-5/98/$0.00+$.50
© 1998 by CRC Press LLC

4.1   CLINICAL ASPECTS

In 1898, it was first appreciated that contact dermatitis had more than one mechanism: irritant and allergic. Most of the investigations this century have focused on the latter. Recent interest in the former mechanism is documented in 1995 textbooks.[2,3] Irritation, or irritant dermatitis, previously considered a monomorphous process, is now understood to be a complex biological syndrome, with a diverse pathophysiology, natural history, and clinical appearance. Thus, the clinical appearance of irritant contact dermatitis varies depending on multiple external ànd internal factors. The actual types, with reference to major characteristics in the clinical appearance, are listed in Table 4.1. This chapter defines the biology of the syndrome in hopes that this will lead to the more efficient development of iontophoresis in humans and animals. As clinical experience with iontophoresis develops, the relationship of irritation from iontophoresis to other forms should be clear.

4.1.1   Acute Irritant Dermatitis (Primary Irritation)

When exposure is sufficient and the offending agent is potent, classic symptoms of acute (primary) skin irritation are seen. Contact with a strong primary irritant is often accidental, and an acute irritant dermatitis is elicited in almost anyone. This classic, acutely developing dermatitis usually heals soon after exposure. In unusual cases the dermatitis may persist for months after exposure, followed by complete resolution.

The availability of the Material Safety Data Sheet and data from the single-application Draize rabbit test, combined with activities of industrial hygienists, toxicologists, dermatologists, and other informed personnel, greatly decreased the frequency of such dermatitis.

4.1.2   Irritant Reaction

Individuals extensively exposed to certain irritants often develop erythematous, chapped skin in the first months of exposure. This irritant reaction[4-6] may be considered a pre-eczematous expression of acute skin irritation. It is frequently seen in

TABLE 4.1
Types of Irritation

Irritation	Onset	Prognosis
Acute primary irritant dermatitis	Acute — often single exposure	Good
Irritant reaction	Acute — often multiple exposure	Good
Delayed acute irritant dermatitis	Delayed — 12 to 24 h or longer	Good
Cumulative irritant contact dermatitis	Slowly developing (weeks to years)	Variable
Traumatic irritant dermatitis	Slowly developing after preceding trauma	Variable
Pustular and acneiform dermatitis	Acute to moderately slowly developing (weeks to months)	Variable
Nonerythematous irritation	Acute to slowly developing	Variable
Friction	Slowly developing	Variable

TABLE 4.2
Chemicals Inducing Delayed, Acute Chemical Irritation

Anthralin	Hydrofluoric acid
Bis (2-chloroethyl)sulfide	Hexanedioldiacrylate
Butanedioldiacrylate	Hydroxypropylacrylate
Dichloro(2-chlorovinyl)arsine	Podophyllin
Epichlorhydrin	Propane sulfone
Ethylene oxide	

repeatedly exposed hairdressers and variable wet work–performing employees. Repeated irritant reactions sometimes lead to contact dermatitis, with good prognosis, although chronic contact dermatitis may also develop. We do not understand what separates the pathophysiology of the low-grade irritant reaction from that of cumulative irritant dermatitis (see below). Once this information becomes available, we may be able to develop interventions to prevent the latter.

4.1.3 DELAYED, ACUTE IRRITANT CONTACT DERMATITIS

Some chemicals produce acute irritation from a single exposure in a delayed manner so that inflammation is not seen until 8 to 24 h or more after exposure.[7,8] Except for the delayed onset, the clinical appearance and course resemble those of acute irritant contact dermatitis. The delayed, acute irritant dermatitis, because of its delayed onset, is often confused with allergic contact dermatitis; appropriately performed and interpreted diagnostic patch tests easily separate the two. Many controls may be required to define those chemicals that are delayed irritants in patch testing (Table 4.2). If this is not done, the delayed onset in the patch may be misinterpreted as allergy rather than delayed onset of acute irritation. This form of irritant dermatitis requires far more investigation. Most of our knowledge comes from patch test observations; use type examples are few.

4.1.4 Cumulative Irritant Dermatitis

When exposure inducing an acute irritant dermatitis is repeated, the dermatitis tends to last longer, and becomes chronic. In cumulative cutaneous irritation, the frequency of exposure is too high in relation to the skin recovery time. Acute irritant skin reaction is not seen in the majority of patients, but mild or moderate, barely visible or invisible skin changes are. Repeated skin exposures and minor reactions lead to a manifest dermatitis when the irritant load exceeds the threshold for visible effects. The development of a cumulative irritant dermatitis was carefully documented by Malten and den Arend[9] and Malten et al.[7] Cumulative irritant dermatitis was called "traumiterative dermatitis" in the older German literature (*traumiterative* = traumas repeating).[10,11] Classic signs are erythema and increasing dryness, followed by hyperkeratosis with frequent cracking and occasional erythema.

Cumulative irritant dermatitis is the most common type of irritant contact dermatitis. This syndrome may develop after days, weeks, or years of subtle exposure to chemical substances. Variation in individual susceptibility increases the multiplicity of clinical findings. Delayed onset and variable attack lead to confusion with allergic contact dermatitis. To rule out allergic etiology, appropriate diagnostic patch testing is indicated. This should be interpreted with the aid of an operational (multifunctional) definition of allergic contact dermatitis.[12,13] This also provides additional integrity to the diagnostic process and decreases the opportunity of misinterpretation of this laboratory test.

4.1.5 Traumatic Irritant Dermatitis

Traumatic irritant dermatitis develops after acute skin trauma. The skin does not heal, but erythema, vesicles and/or vesicopapules, and scaling appear. The clinical course later resembles nummular (coin-shaped) dermatitis. This may occur after burns or lacerations and after acute irritant dermatitis; it may be compounded by a concurrent allergen exposure.[14] The healing period is generally prolonged.

Often these patients are considered to have a factitial dermatitis because of a healing phase followed by exacerbation. Although factitial aspects may occur in some patients, this peculiar form of irritation appears to be a disease *sui generis*. Its chronicity and recalcitrance to therapy provides a challenge to both patient and physician. We have no information explaining why the occasional patient develops this phenomenon, and how this patient differs from the general population.

4.1.6 Pustular and Acneiform Irritant Dermatitis

Pustular and acneiform irritant dermatitis may develop from exposure to cosmetics, skin care agents, metals, oils and greases, tar, asphalt, chlorinated naphthalenes, and polyhalogenated naphthalenes. Certain substances have a capacity to elicit these reactions,[15,16] and even allergic reactions may sometimes be pustular or follicular.[17] In occupational exposure, only a minority of subjects develop pustular or acneiform dermatitis. Thus, the development of this type of irritant contact dermatitis appears to be dependent on both constitutional and chemical factors. Wahlberg and Maibach[18] developed an animal model for its investigation. This special form of irritant dermatitis has not received adequate investigation.

4.1.7 NONERYTHEMATOUS IRRITATION

In the early stages of skin irritation, subtle skin damage may occur without visible inflammation. As a correlate of nonvisible irritation, objectively registered alterations in the damaged epidermis have been reported.[19-21] It is customary in Japan to screen new chemicals, cosmetics, and textiles for subtle signs of stratum corneum damage, employing replicas of stratum corneum (the Kawai method). Consumer dissatisfaction with many chemicals may result from exposure to this low-grade irritation; thus, the patient feels more than the physician observes.

4.1.8 SENSORY (SUBJECTIVE) IRRITATION

Sensory (subjective) irritation is experienced by some individuals ("stingers") in contact with certain chemicals.[21,22] Itching, stinging, or tingling is experienced, for example, from skin contact with lactic acid, a model for nonvisible cutaneous irritation. The threshold for this reaction varies among subjects, independent of susceptibility to other irritation types. The quality as well as the concentration of the exposing agent, is also important, and neural pathways may be contributory, but the pathomechanism is unknown. Some sensory irritation may be subclinical contact urticaria. Screening raw ingredients and final formulations in the guinea pig ear swelling test[23] or the human forehead assay allows us to minimize the amount of subclinical contact urticaria.

Although sensory irritation has a neural component (being blocked by local anesthetics), Lammintausta et al.[21] suggest that the blood vessel may be more responsive in stingers than nonstingers.[24] At least 10% of women complain of stinging with certain facial products; thus, further work is needed to develop a strategy to overcome this type of discomfort. Further investigations on progress of sensory anti-irritants is promising (Hahn, G., personal communication).

4.1.9 LOCALIZATION OF IRRITANT CONTACT DERMATITIS

Cua et al.[25] summarize regional anatomic variation in relation to susceptibility to irritation.

4.2 EXTERNAL FACTORS

4.2.1 IRRITANTS

Many chemicals qualify as irritants when the exposing dose is high.[26] Molecular size, ionization, polarization, fat solubility, and other factors that are important in skin penetration are also important in cutaneous irritation.[27] The threshold of strength and quality of irritation depends on the physicochemical properties of the substance. Temperature may be important, with warm temperatures generally more damaging than cool[28]; e.g., warm citral perfume produced more irritation than citral at lower temperature.

4.2.2 Exposure

The absorbed dose may vary when the substance is suspended in different vehicles.[29-32] The solubility of the irritant in the vehicle and the inherent irritancy of the vehicle have an impact on each reaction.[33] The effective tissue dose depends on concentration, volume, application time, and duration on and in the skin. Long exposure time and large volume may increase penetration. Thus, greater response may be expected. If exposure is repeated, the recovery from previous exposure(s) affects the subsequent response. Sometimes a shorter, repeated exposure leads to a lengthened recovery period.[9] This was demonstrated in experimental studies with dimethyl sulfoxide (DMSO). Intermittent application during 1 day leads to a different response as compared with one application.[34] These experimental observations are consistent with the multiple clinical appearances of cumulative irritant dermatitis.

4.2.3 Multiple Simultaneous Exposure

Simultaneous or subsequent exposure may lead to an additive effect and increased reaction, although each chemical alone would elicit only a minor reaction, or none. On the other hand, subsequent exposure may lead to a decreased response. For instance, exposure to a detergent and then to a soap led to a response less than exposure to a detergent alone. The detergent was washed away by the subsequent soap exposure.[35] Patil et al.[36] observed that repeated exposure of skin (*in vivo*) to sodium lauryl sulfate (SLS) leads to a prolonged damage to the skin in that region and the skin does not come back to normal even 12 days after exposure to the irritant. An "overlap phenomenon" (exaggerated reaction in the adjacent region of the pre-exposed site) was reported using bioengineering methods. Studies on rat skin[37] have also demonstrated residual levels of SLS in the skin 1 week after exposure to SLS. SLS tends to accumulate into the epidermis after repeated exposure and is not cleared away by the dermal supply. A radial spread of this compound was observed up to ~0.75 cms from the site of application in a classic 24-hour study.[38]

The outcome of multiple, subsequent, or simultaneous exposures is sometimes unexpected[39] and rules must be sought.[40] In any instance, any skin pretreatment prior to iontophoresis should be evaluated for its irritation-potentiating effects.

4.2.4 Other Irritation Sources

Physical trauma from friction often facilitates the harmful effects of a chemical irritant. Repeated microtrauma and friction typically lead to dry, hyperkeratotic, and abraded skin.[41] Although physical irritation alone may produce irritant dermatitis, the additive effect with chemical exposure may lead to irritant contact dermatitis. Corresponding impact is seen with other physical irritants.

Quantification of physical trauma from friction and differences in individual susceptibility to friction are expected to lead to appropriate interventions to decrease such damage.

TABLE 4.3
Effect of Duration of Occlusion
on Percutaneous Absorption
of Malathion in Humans

Duration (h)	Absorption (%)
0[a]	9.6
0.5	7.3
1	12.7
2	16.6
4	24.2
8	38.8
24	62.8

[a] Immediate wash with soap and water.

Source: Feldmann, R.J. and Maibach, H.I., Report to the Federal Working Group on pest management from the Task Group on Occupational Exposure to Pesticides, Appendix B, pp. 120–127, 1974.

4.2.5 ENVIRONMENTAL FACTORS

Low environmental humidity enhances irritability: skin tests with irritants produce more and stronger reactions in winter when the weather is cool, windy, and dry.[42] It also produces variable irritation symptoms: itching and erythema associated with whealing or erythema and scaling.[43,44] Occlusion often enhances penetration and increases acute irritation[45] (Table 4.3). Thus, skin reactions frequently become stronger when the chemical is applied under occlusion, providing a humid environment that minimizes evaporation and makes the stratum corneum more permeable.

4.3 PREDISPOSING FACTORS

4.3.1 METHODOLOGICAL ASPECTS

Although irritant contact dermatitis accounts for most occupational skin diseases and although many nonoccupational eczemas are exclusively or partially induced by irritation, in-depth investigation of irritant contact dermatitis is infrequent. Epidemiological studies have identified many important irritants, and some information is available about subjects who appear vulnerable to irritant dermatitis in occupational circumstances that induce dermatitis. Detergents and soaps are considered principal causes of occupational irritant dermatitis. However, in controlled experimental trials, this implied harmful effect of soap has not always been documented.[46-50] Correspondingly, with evaluation of patch test reactions to detergents by direct visualization, individual differences in irritant reactivity were not documented in healthy skin. Only those subjects with a concurrent eczema reacted more

TABLE 4.4
Bioengineering Techniques Used in the Evaluation of Cutaneous Irritation

Technique	Measured Skin Function	Advantages	Disadvantages
Laser Doppler velocimetry	Velocity of the moving erythrocytes with blood flow	Slight, pre-erythema	Does not measure nonerythematous irritation
Evaporimeter	Transepidermal water exchange evaluated	Epidermal damage evaluated; easy to use	Visible erythema Inflammation contributes but does not directly correlate Standardized environmental circumstances important
Ultrasound	Skin thickness	Edematous inflammation measured	Minimal correlation with visible erythema or epidermal damage
Impedance, conductance and capacitance	Skin hydration	Correlation with epidermal damage	
Colorimeter	Skin colors	Correlation with erythema, inflammation	Correlates with the amount of pigment, too. Minimal correlation with epidermal damage and other nonerythematous inflammation

strongly.[21,51] Bioengineering methods now make it possible to quantitate minor differences in cutaneous reactivity.

Nonvisible cutaneous changes are measurable with various methods in which different aspects of skin function are quantitated. Table 4.4 lists available and useful instrumentation with reference to the measured physicochemical parameters. Documented are alterations in impedance,[52] transepidermal water loss (TEWL), dielectric characteristics,[53] conductance and resistance,[54] blood flow velocity,[55] and skin thickness.[56] Skin pH[57] and O_2 resistance and CO_2 effusion rates[58,59] are further measurable skin changes in skin irritation. Measurements of these variables often show poor correlation with each other, probably because these methods give information about different aspects of cutaneous irritation and skin function. Recent textbooks provide in-depth overviews of utilization of these methods in dermatopharmacology, toxicology, and physiology.[3,60-62]

In addition to patch testing with irritants accompanied by visual scoring, alkali resistance and alkali neutralization capacity have been evaluated by using ammonium hydroxide applications. Their capacity to reflect individual susceptibility appears to be limited or minimal[63] and their value is questioned.

Wilhelm et al.[64] utilized sodium hydroxide to produce transepidermal water loss as a measure of skin damage. This assay shows a high correlation between subjects developing increased water loss after application of sodium hydroxide and a propensity

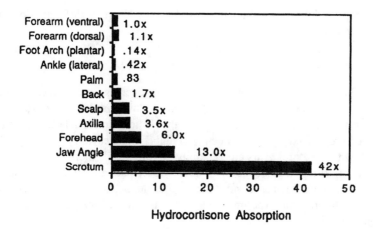

Hydrocortisone Absorption

FIGURE 4.1   Anatomic regional variation of percutaneous absorption in humans. (Adapted from Feldmann and Maibach.[67])

for SLS damage. This simple approach may provide a first step toward a preemployment test for irritant dermatitis potential.

Individual susceptibility to chemicals has been studied by documenting skin reactivity to model irritants. The intensity of the wheal created by DMSO, the time required to raise a blister (minimal blistering time, or MBT) after cutaneous application of aluminum hydroxide solution, and reactivity to SLS are examples of objective methods that have been used.[65,66] Stinging (sensory irritation) occurs with certain test substances (e.g., lactic acid), and clinical experiments provide some information about individual susceptibility.[22]

Despite important steps taken in the investigation of the pathogenesis of irritant contact dermatitis, no experimental design has proved entirely successful for the clinical evaluation of individual susceptibility.

4.3.2   REGIONAL ANATOMIC DIFFERENCES

Anatomic differences in the exposure site are important. Because skin permeability is variable in different skin sites, being generally greatest in thin skin areas,[67-71] corresponding association between permeability, skin thickness, and skin irritation is expected, but direct correlation is lacking (Figure 4.1). Regional variation has been studied comparing the whealing response — a variation of immediate irritation — to DMSO and measuring differences in MBT after topical ammonium hydroxide application in different skin sites.[22]

Both tests showed the mandibular area to be most reactive, followed by the upper back, forearm, lower leg, and palm. With DMSO whealing, the forehead was more sensitive than the back, the antecubital area reaction preceded that of the rest of the upper extremity, and the wrist was more sensitive than the leg.

In patch testing, the irritant benzalkonium chloride and several allergens produced maximal reactivity in the upper back,[72] an observation recently extended to the middle scapula.[73] The greater reactivity may be related to pressure in this area when sleeping.[74,75] Certain "inherent" differences between different skin sites in irritation reactivity may also exist.

4.3.3 AGE

The threshold for skin irritation is believed to be decreased in babies, who develop dermatitis from irritation that does not occur in adult skin.[78,79] Except for structural and functional immaturity of infant's skin, other factors (intestinal *Candida albicans,* completed breast feeding, low frequency of diaper changes) are contributory.[80] Children below the age of 8 years are generally believed to be more susceptible to skin irritation.[81-83] Irritation susceptibility gradually decreases after this age. Maibach and Boisits[84] define this database; unfortunately, despite extensive chemical exposure of infants and children, our experimental evidence is lacking because of methodological problems and limited data.

Skin problems commonly occur in the elderly.[85] In a majority of cutaneous symptoms, cutaneous irritation is contributory. Elderly subjects may develop reactions to skin irritants less sharply and more slowly than younger individuals.[86,87] A corresponding alteration occurs with regard to cutaneous reactivity to allergens. With ammonium hydroxide skin tests, older subjects had a shorter reaction time (MBT), whereas the time needed to develop a tense blister was longer,[88] and a longer time was needed for the resorption of a wheal elicited by saline injection.[89] That aspect of responsiveness related to percutaneous penetration has been reviewed by Roskos and Maibach.[90]

Age-associated alterations in skin reactivity may be related to altered cutaneous permeation, although contradictory results have been reported.[91-95] Alterations in structural lipids[96] and in cell composition[97] and renewal[98,99] are reported in association with structural alteration.[100,101] Thus, age-associated alterations in cutaneous reactivity are expected; however, the subject requires more investigation.

4.3.4 RACE

It is difficult to compare irritant reactions in white and black skin, although black skin less frequently seems (to the naked eye) to develop irritation from chemicals eliciting irritant reactions in white skin.[102,103] When blood flow velocity is altered in an irritant reaction, the reaction is measurable with laser Doppler velocimetry (LDV). Observations in experimental studies using LDV support *increased* reactivity to a detergent in black subjects[19] (Table 4.5).

Black skin has higher electrical resistance than does Caucasoid skin.[104] Because of this characteristic, it may have increased resistance to irritants that themselves often lower electrical skin resistance. Structural differences are reported, too, such as difference in skin reactivity to irritants when minimal perceptible erythema was registered.[102] Black skin, however, needs more stripping for the removal of stratum corneum.[105] With methacholine-induced erythema and flare response, black skin appear to be less reactive than white.[106]

Clinical experiments suggest that black skin has differences in the modulation of irritation reactivity as compared with white skin.[19] It may be reflected in certain

TABLE 4.5
Laser Doppler Velocimetry (LDV)
Values in Blacks and Whites

LDV (mV)	Preoccluded		
	0.5%[a]		2.0%
Whites	73.6 ± 34	$p < 0.01$	179 ± 128
Blacks	58 ± 25	$p < 0.01$	234 ± 194

Note: p values refer to the comparison between 0.5% and 2% SLS concentration.

[a] $p < 0.04$ for blacks vs. whites.

aspects of the multifactoral development of skin irritation, which is, however, still inadequately understood. Cutaneous erythema induced by methacholine injections was compared in Warain Indians, Tibetans, and Caucasians. Caucasians reacted to the greatest degree,[107] and associations between skin irritation and cholinergic reactivity may exist.[19] Berardesca and Maibach[108] provide additional details.

4.3.5 GENDER

The incidence of clinical irritant contact dermatitis — most often located in the hands — is higher in females than in males.[11,109,110] Because of this clinical observation, susceptibility to skin irritation has been related to female skin, which also seems to elicit more tape irritation.[111,112] Skin tests with surfactants, however, have not experimentally documented a difference.[113,114] The increased occurrence of irritant contact dermatitis may be related to the more extensive exposure to irritants and wet work. A minimal relationship between gender and constitutional skin irritability is supported by the fact that the female preponderance in the irritant contact dermatitis populations does not hold true for all geographic areas.[115] Socioeconomic factors may be responsible.

4.3.6 GENETICS

Interindividual variation based on genetic constitutional differences has been demonstrated.[51,65] When patch test reactivity to common irritants was compared between monozygotic and dizygotic twins with control subjects, the highest degree of concordance was demonstrated for the monozygotic twin pairs.[116]

Susceptibility to sunlight has been associated with vulnerability to chemical irritants. Sun-sensitive skin and low minimal erythema dose (MED) appears to correlate with high cutaneous irritability.[117,118] Marked interindividual variation in skin reactivity has been demonstrated with the alkali resistance test, although the relevance to clinical irritant reactivity is minor.[63]

In a large series, individual skin irritability varied for different chemical irritants when reactions were evaluated with visual scoring.[51] These results were confirmed by Czerwinska-Dihm and Rudzki.[119] Both sets of data support the simultaneous influence of the quality of irritant, individual susceptibility, and multiple environmental factors. For experimental studies, certain model irritants are needed; however, the results may not be generalizable.

A test battery consisting of DMSO reactivity, blistering susceptibility to ammonium hydroxide, and SLS reactivity was found useful.[65] Unfortunately, it is too complicated to be used in clinical practice for preemployment testing.

Newer bioengineering test methods show great interindividual variation. For example, TEWL, which is easy to measure, reflects important components of detergent-induced irritation. In the evaluation of individual irritant reactivity, however, repeated follow-up measurements are needed, because baseline values do not necessarily reflect the reactivity when irritation is produced.

4.3.7 PREVIOUS AND PREEXISTING SKIN DISEASES

Subjects with a previous or present atopic dermatitis have an increased susceptibility to develop irritant dermatitis.[109,120] Ichthyosis vulgaris is sometimes seen in association with atopic dermatitis; in ichthyosis vulgaris, patients' irritant reactivity has been shown to be increased to alkali irritants.[121] The increased general cutaneous irritability related to atopic dermatitis[122] could not be demonstrated with regular patch tests when skin irritants were used.[123,124]

Reduced capacity to bind water has been related to atopic skin,[125] which in noneczematous sites demonstrates greater TEWL than does nonatopic skin. Stratum corneum water content may even be increased.[126-128] An increased water loss was induced with detergent patch tests in atopic skin.[20] Itchy and dry atopic skin has been connected with an increased risk for developing hand dermatitis.[109,129] However, certain atopic subjects with rhinitis or asthma have normal, nonirritable skin, and an itchy and dryness-prone skin may be seen in some nonatopic subjects. Accurate objective tools are not available to evaluate the atopic cutaneous characteristics or atopic skin diathesis.

Seborrheic skin has not been shown to possess increased susceptibility to skin irritants; reports and interpretations are contradictory.[130-132] Clinical experience suggests that some increased irritability is associated with a seborrheic constitution in certain subjects. This may be true in certain geographic areas, where environmental humidity is low in the winter in relation to the cold temperatures.

Different methods have been used in studies on skin irritability in individuals with psoriasis. Those studies revealed decreased and increased irritant reactivity[118,133-135] when anthralin (dithranol) irritancy was the main interest. Psoriatic skin is particularly irritable in certain individuals,[136] and the development of psoriatic lesions in irritation sites (Koebner phenomenon) is often seen.

In the presence of eczema, the threshold for skin irritation is decreased.[51,137-139] A whole-body examination of employees sometimes reveals nummular lesions or other constitutional eczema symptoms. Such a clinical finding may suggest an increased skin irritability in different locations. Pompholyx (dyshidrosis) type dermatitis is harmful. As a constitutional eczema, it probably increases skin irritability in general. These patients often have difficulty wearing gloves, since pompholyx is made worse by occlusion.

A history of contact dermatitis may be important when susceptibility to irritant contact dermatitis is evaluated.[34,140] Although increased irritability has been hard to demonstrate,[34,51] further improvement of methodological equipment and techniques in bioengineering should make this possible.

Recently, skin reactivity was found to be decreased in patients with X-linked recessive icthyosis.[141]

4.3.8 SYSTEMIC SKIN DISEASE — ATOPIC DERMATITIS

On the basis of dermatological clinical experience, patients with atopic dermatitis have irritable skin manifested by reactivity to all types of irritants.[120] Since facial dermatitis and hand dermatitis are common in atopic dermatitis, it appears that irritation is an important factor. In wet work, for example, in which exposure to water, detergents, or other chemicals is frequent or continuous, the subjects with a history of atopic dermatitis develop hand dermatitis more often than those without a history of atopic symptoms.[20,129,140] The studies also suggest that atopic subjects with dry, itchy skin have skin problems more often than nonatopic subjects in environments where exposure to irritants is extensive, although they would not have histories of manifest skin effects.[129] In these subjects, the threshold level for cutaneous irritation from repeated irritant attacks appears intermediate between those with atopic dermatitis and those with a nonatopic constitution.

Cutaneous irritability in atopic subjects shows considerable clinical variation. The degree is dependent on the number of characteristics in the skin that make the skin particularly prone to develop cutaneous irritation. The scale is wide. Simultaneously, many atopic subjects — some 30 to 40% of those with only mucosal symptoms — have normal skin without demonstrable susceptibilities.

4.4 EXPERIMENTAL STUDIES IN IRRITANT DERMATITIS SYNDROME

4.4.1 EXPERIMENTAL IRRITANT DERMATITIS

Irritant dermatitis is induced with patch test technique and read on the basis of visual scoring of elicited irritant reactions of variable degree. The strength of one reaction does not usually predict reactivity to other irritants.[51] The alkali resistance test as a predictive test for irritability has not proved reliable.[63]

In human experiments, visible reactions to different irritants — whealing from DMSO contact, blister formation from ammonium hydroxide, and eczematous reactions after contact with SLS, alkyldimethyl benzyl ammonium chloride, croton oil, or kerosene — have suggested that some part of individual variation in cutaneous irritant reactivity may be predictable.[120] Hyper- and hyporeacting groups may be recognizable to some extent.

Investigators have worked on methodological improvements in irritant dermatitis studies, because visual assessment measures mainly erythema and edema and is subjective.

Besides the limitations in qualitative aspects, the reliability of observed and visually quantitated results may be limited. Tools employed in clinical experiments are the laser Doppler flowmeter, evaporimeter, micrometers, and ultrasonography. Skin impedance and water content have been measured and replica systems developed to qualify and quantify reactions.[53] In experimental irritant dermatitis studies, certain model irritants, usually detergents, were used. SLS is the model surfactant used most frequently.[66] Note that it represents mainly two types of irritant dermatitis (acute and cumulative), and should not be assumed to represent all types and causes of this complex syndrome. It induces epidermal damage as well as visible erythematous irritation and thus is a useful model irritant for such experiments.

The laser Doppler flowmeter gives information about cutaneous circulatory changes associated with erythematous irritation. Results obtained with laser Doppler generally correlate with visible changes.[55,142,143] This method appears slightly more sensitive than the naked eye in evaluating erythema, which is often correlated with the amount of epidermal damage.[21,34]

Edema may sometimes interfere with measurements, and thus reactions with associated edema yield lower flowmeter values, although irritation-induced reaction in skin vasculature is apparent.[21] Nonerythematous irritation cannot be detected with this method.

The evaporimeter is a practical tool for the measurement of transepidermal loss.[143] Cumulative irritation leads to increased TEWL.[34] Increased irritation from more concentrated irritants leads to greater increase in TEWL, although no erythema is seen. These alterations can be demonstrated before visible changes appear. TEWL often increases in association with erythematous irritation,[34,144] which makes this method useful in studies of more acute irritant responses. The recovery of epidermis after irritant attacks has been demonstrated with gradually normalizing TEWL values. Evaporimeter measurements are quick; measurement can be registered in minutes. But the resting time needed before individual values can be evaluated has to be 20 to 30 min, since nonsweating baseline values must first be obtained. Environmental circumstances (temperature and humidity) must be standardized.[145] For evaluations of individual reactivity, repeated values have to be followed up, since individual baseline values are different. On the other hand, baseline values for an individual subject show day-to-day variation. TEWL measurements still need standardization and improvement before this tool is useful for routine clinical purposes.

The measurement of skin electrical impedance and water content provides further means of studying cutaneous hydration.[52-54] Impedance measurement is based on the facilitated current conduction in stratum corneum related to the ionic movements of hydrates. Stratum corneum water content is assessed by means of a microwave dielectric probe.

Future efforts will be directed to developing these methods for practical purposes. Studies of the mechanisms of irritant contact dermatitis on the cellular and biochemical level will reveal new aspects to this syndrome. Increasing knowledge about mediators[146,147] and cell interactions[148,149] will also help us to understand this multifactorial clinical problem.

4.4.2 CONCOMITANT DISEASE

Generalized wasting and debilitation in patients with advanced carcinoma have been associated with decreased skin reactivity to croton oil and dinitrochlorobenzene (DNCB).[150] Decreased reactivity to croton oil[151] and increased susceptibility to alkali[121] were reported in patients with ichthyosis vulgaris. Other investigators noted increased reactivity to phenol[152] but decreased reactivity to croton oil[153] on the depigmented skin in patients with vitiligo. The literature on patch test reactions to irritants in the presence of eczema is conflicting. This subject has been partly clarified by Bjornberg,[51] who showed that an increased susceptibility to irritants may be demonstrated in eczematous patients with some but *not all* irritants. Susceptibility to irritation has also been correlated with the extent of the eczema. Patients with *localized* hand eczema had increased reactivity to SLS; patients with *generalized* eczema had increased reactivity to four additional irritants (croton oil, trichloroacetic acid, mercury bichloride, and sapo kalinus). Bjornberg et al.[154] further demonstrated that patients with healed hand eczema have no greater susceptibility to irritants than noneczematous controls. The type of eczema may also influence the response to irritants. Skog[123] showed an increased incidence of primary irritant reactions to pentadecylcatechol in patients with preexisting allergic contact eczema but not in patients with preexisting irritant eczema or atopic dermatitis. Although clinical observations have suggested that individuals with atopic dermatitis or atopic diathesis are more susceptible to skin irritation, experimental proof is lacking.

4.4.3 NEUROLOGICAL INFLUENCE

Neurological factors may influence cutaneous reactivity. Biberstein[155] reported an increased inflammatory response to mustard oil on sympathectomized ears in rabbits, compared with nonsympathectomized contralateral control ears. Others reported decreased reactivity to phenol in areas of peripheral paralysis but increased reactivity to phenol in areas of central paralysis,[156] decreased reactivity to tincture of iodine in areas of peripheral anesthesia,[157] and a generalized increase in reactivity in areas of peripheral neuritis.[153]

The nervous system is obviously involved in the subjective response to irritants. A specific somatosensory receptor, selectively stimulated by certain irritants (e.g., lacrimators), has been identified in cat skin.[158]

4.4.4 MEDICATION (PHARMACOLOGY)

Corticosteroids in sufficient dose administered either topically or systemically may suppress subsequent irritant responses to croton oil,[159] but not to turpentine or cantharidin.[160] In general, there appears to be a limiting dose of systemically administered corticosteroid below which the inflammatory response is not inhibited. Although there is not universal agreement, the limiting dose appears to be in the range of 15 mg of prednisone or equivalent.[161] Antihistamines in any dose probably do not impair responses to irritants. No data exist on the cutaneous response to irritants in patients with Addison's or Cushing's disease. Funk and Maibach[162] have reviewed this area in depth.

4.5   PREDICTIVE IRRITANCY TESTING

Predictive irritancy testing involves specific tests for the irritant potential of individual chemicals as well as tests for individual susceptibility to irritation.

4.5.1   PREDICTIVE TESTING FOR CHEMICAL IRRITANT POTENTIAL

Predictive testing is widely performed to determine the irritant potential of various chemicals. The most popular methods are bioassays with human or animal subjects. Most procedures employ a single application of a test substance, with evaluation of the response in 24 to 48 h. The oldest of these assays is the Draize rabbit test, in which test substances are applied for 24 h under occlusion to abraded and nonabraded skin. While this procedure detects severe irritants for human skin, it is unsatisfactory for mild to moderate irritants.[163] Numerous modifications adaptable to special situations have been developed; a National Research Council[164] special publication discusses the principles and practices involved.

Because of species variability, correlation of irritancy studies of animal skin with human skin has not been entirely satisfactory. A rabbit cumulative irritancy test has been described that compares favorably with a cumulative human irritancy assay.[165,166]

Bioassays involving human subjects are patterned after those involving animal models. Frosch and Kligman[167] introduced a chamber scarification test, which enhances the capacity to detect mild irritants. The forearm is scarified in a crisscross pattern; the suspected irritant is applied to this area in a large aluminum chamber once daily for 3 days.

To date, bioassays have utilized visible degrees of erythema and edema as indices of irritancy; this method is simple and convenient. The development of physical techniques for measuring subtle degrees of noninflammatory skin damage has improved our understanding of this area. Skin permeability to water vapor (TEWL) was the first physical measurement to be used for this purpose. Early investigations established that chemicals that provoked inflammation increased TEWL.[168-170] Malten and Thiele[171] subsequently showed that increases in TEWL occurred *before* visible inflammation when ionic, polar, water-soluble substances (e.g., sodium hydroxide, soaps, detergents) were used as irritants. Malten and den Arend[9] showed that an unionized, polar irritant (DMSO) did not provoke increased water vapor loss until visible inflammation had already occurred. Similarly, two unionized nonpolar (water-insoluble) irritants, hexanediol diacrylate and butanediol diacrylate, did not provoke increased skin water vapor loss until visible inflammation occurred.[7] Thus, TEWL measurements may detect the irritant capacity of certain chemicals in the absence of visible inflammation, but possibly only for ionizable, polar, water-soluble substances.

Measurements of the electrical impedance (resistance) of human skin also detect subtle degrees of skin damage before skin inflammation occurs.[52] This method has the advantage over water loss measurements that it is capable of detecting subtle changes produced by unionizable or nonpolar substances as well as ionizable, polar ones.[7]

Measurements of carbon dioxide emission from human skin have been developed.[171] Rates of carbon dioxide emission from irritated skin increase roughly in proportion to the degree of irritation.[172]

Electrolyte flux through the skin barrier may be measured with the aid of ion-specific skin electrodes.[59,173] Measurements of chloride ion flux through psoriatic or eczematous skin indicate that, despite the dramatic increases in permeability to water vapor, the electrolyte barrier remains relatively intact.[59] Chloride ion flux may provide another noninflammatory index of cutaneous irritation. A potassium ion electrode has been of value in quantifying potassium flux post damage.[174]

4.5.2 PREDICTIVE TESTING FOR SUSCEPTIBILITY TO IRRITATION

The ability to predict which individuals are more prone to irritant skin reactions has practical significance as a preemployment screening test. The ability of the skin to neutralize solutions of sodium hydroxide was first proposed as a screening test for susceptibility to irritation by Gross et al.[175] Bjornberg[51] reviewed previous attempts to predict general susceptibility by determining irritant responses to selected irritants. He was unable to corroborate early claims that inability to neutralize alkaline solutions, decreased resistance to alkaline irritation, or that increased susceptibility to common experimental irritants could be used to predict susceptibility to irritations in a preemployment setting.

Frosch and Kligman,[88] using the length of time to slight blister formation after experimental exposure to ammonium hydroxide as a predictive index, found that short times were highly correlated with the intensity of inflammation produced by irritating concentrations of SLS. They also found that patients with atopic dermatitis (who were presumably more susceptible to irritation) had shorter times to blister formation than controls.[176]

4.6 IN VITRO ASSAYS

This rapidly developing area has been extensively documented by Rougier et al.[177]

4.7 HISTOLOGY, HISTOPATHOLOGY, AND PATHOLOGY

Contact dermatitis, eczema, and eczematous lesions are imprecise terms in dermatologic histology. Irritant contact dermatitis cannot be characterized on the basis of histological findings. The histology is different in acute and chronic contact dermatitis. The degree and severity of the dermatitis and the interval between the onset and the actual time of biopsy influence the histological findings.

If the acute irritant or toxic skin reaction is strong, vesicles may be seen. In the vesicle, a mixture of neutrophils and lymphocytes is seen. In initial acute irritant contact dermatitis, dermal changes may be absent or minimal. Dermal infiltrates appear and increase during the first day of the developing dermatitis. The cell infiltrates in irritant and allergic contact dermatitis are not significantly or diagnostically different. In chronic irritant contact dermatitis, scaling, hyperkeratosis, and lichenification are apparent in older skin lesions, often resembling neurodermatitis.

In immunohistological studies, identical composition of peripheral T lymphocytes, associated with peripheral HLA-DR (histocompatibility locus A) positive macrophages and Langerhans cells, is seen in irritant and allergic contact dermatitis.[178,179] In the lymphocyte population, helper/inducer lymphocytes exceed the number of T-suppression/cytotoxic cells.[178,180] In irritant contact dermatitis, keratinocytes have been demonstrated to express major histocompatibility complex (MHC) class II antigens concerned with the antigen presentation and the elicitation of the T-lymphocyte-dependent immune response.[149] These antigens were expressed by the keratinocytes in both allergic and irritant contact dermatitis.

The inflammatory cell response has also been characterized in guinea pigs treated with toxic croton oil application or repeated SLS applications. In both reactions monocyte counts were increased, even as compared with an allergic reaction. The heterogeneous monocyte group, however, consisted of lymphocytes, fibroblasts, and monocytes. Only a minority of basophils was seen, less than in allergic contact reactions. Mast cells were also slightly increased, suggesting some association between nonimmunologic contact urticaria and an acute irritant contact reaction.[181]

Irritants, such as surfactants, removed skin lipids and keratins. The mechanisms of inflammation in the development of irritant contact dermatitis are still poorly understood. In laboratory animals, the importance of the function and inflammation mediators of different cell types is appreciated, and certain preliminary observations have been reported in constructed experimental designs. For example, SLS and alkyl dimethyl benzammonium chloride (ADBC) were shown to enhance the migration of polymorphonuclear leukocytes. A corresponding inhibition was induced by leukotriene B4; that is, SLS and ADBC also induced the secretion of preformed mediators, such as histamine and lysozymal enzyme β-G from the cells.[148] Wide variation in the inhibitory response was documented for cutaneous inflammation elicited by different irritants, whether induction was by histamine antagonists, prostaglandin and kinin synthesis inhibitors, or neutropenia-inducing agents.[182]

The importance of leukotrienes in irritant contact dermatitis appears evident,[147] and a peptidoleukotriene antagonist and an antagonist of platelet-activating factor (PAF) were documented to be less effective in irritant contact dermatitis than in the allergic type, suggesting that cytotoxic effects predominate in irritant contact dermatitis.[146]

A corresponding interpretation was made based on the observation that the lipoxygenesis pathway is enhanced in irritant contact dermatitis, whereas it is inhibited in allergic contact dermatitis.[183]

4.7.1 Ulceration

Ulcerative lesions can develop from skin contact with strong acids or strong alkalies. Calcium oxide and calcium hydroxide, sodium hydroxide, sodium metasilicate and sodium silicate, potassium cyanide, and trisodium phosphate may induce strong cutaneous irritation with ulcerations. Chrome ulcers are the most common type of cutaneous ulcers induced by irritation of dichromates. Compounds of beryllium, arsenic, or cadmium are also capable of inducing strong irritation and ulcers.

Solvents such as acrylonitrile and carbon bisulfide as well as gaseous ethylene oxide are examples of contactants that may induce ulceration in certain occupations. Cutaneous ulcerations develop from the direct corrosive and necrotizing effect of the chemical on the living tissue. Exposed areas, where both friction and chemical irritation are associated, are most susceptible for ulcers; minor preceding trauma in the exposed skin increases the risk. The ulcerations tend to be deeper, with an undermined thickened border, and the exudate under the covering crusts predisposes to infection. The treatment for ulcers is usually conservative, with dressings, powders, and different coverings according to the phase of healing. In some cases, such as beryllium ulcerations, excision has been recommended.

4.7.2 GRANULOMAS

Cutaneous granulomas are considered a variant of irritant or/and allergic contact dermatitis when caused by a biologically inactive substance inoculated into the skin. A granuloma appears as a focal, tumid lesion persisting chronically in its primary site. It is subjectively symptomless. Macrophages respond with phagocytosis to the foreign body inoculation, and even giant cells may be seen.[184]

In clinical occupational dermatitis, the development is generally due to an accidental foreign body inoculation of hard and sharp plant parts, hairs, or different hard keratin animal parts into the skin of the employee. Powders, lead, and metals, such as metallic mercury, beryllium, and silica, are examples of substances that elicit toxic skin granulomas.[185] Infectious granulomas may be caused by deep fungi, bacteria, or parasites. In these cases, inflammation and macrophage response, with phagocytic secretory and mixed function macrophages, are seen.

Examining occupational dermatologists should keep the possibility of irritation granuloma in mind when studying and performing biopsy on this type of lesion; they should remind the histopathologist to utilize the special maneuvers needed to demonstrate possible foreign bodies. Special stains, electron microscopy, and the use of polarized light are often useful.[186]

4.7.3 HARDENING

Extensive and repeated exposure often produces an increased resistance to further irritation in the course of weeks or months. The importance of interindividual variation in the development of hardening may be even greater than the threshold level for cutaneous irritation, since the individual capacity to recover from previous attacks is a factor. The developed resistance or hardening is specific to the substance inducing it. It is restricted to the affected skin area; certain subjects appear to be unable to develop hardening. Relatively short periods away from work decrease the resistance, again increasing the vulnerability for irritant contact dermatitis after holidays. The "hardened" skin appears coarse, thickened, and somewhat lichenified. Increased skin thickness may play a role in the development of hardening. Skin thickening was evident in the experimental hardening state in guinea pigs.[187] Unfortunately, the main biological mechanisms are unknown.

Repeated UV exposures also increase the capacity to resist irritation in the skin. This effect appears to be nonspecific.[188] Repeated UV exposures are therapeutic, followed by a period of hardening in the treatment of subacute or chronic irritant contact dermatitis. When the acute phase of an irritant contact dermatitis is over and relapses are expected, repeated UV exposures may elicit nonspecific "desensitization" in the skin, increasing the capacity to avoid relapses. Alterations at the cellular level, in cell surface proteins, and in the releasability of inflammatory mediators probably are important in the therapeutic benefit achieved by UV therapies of irritant contact dermatitis.

4.7.4 METHODS FOR DEFINING IONTOPHORESIS-RELATED IRRITANT DERMATITIS

Camel et al.[189,190] have proposed methodology to quantify iontophoresis-induced irritant dermatitis, utilizing bioengineering methodology as an addition to the human eye and finger for quantification.

GENERAL READING

Elsner, P., Maibach, H.I., Eds. 1995. *Irritant Dermatitis,* S. Karger, New York.
Elsner, P., Wahlberg, J., Maibach, H.I., 1996. *Prevention of Contact Dermatitis,* Karger, New York.
Marzulli, F., Maibach, H.I., Eds. 1995. *Dermatoxicology,* 5th ed., Taylor and Francis, Washington, D.C.
Menne, T., Maibach, H.I., Eds. 1994. *Hand Eczema,* CRC Press, Boca Raton, FL.
Rougier, A., Goldberg, A.M., Maibach, H.I., 1994. *In Vitro Skin Toxicology: Irritation, Phototoxicity, Sensitization.* (Alternative Methods in Toxocology Series, Vol. 10), Mary Ann Liebert, Inc., New York.
Van der Valk, P., Maibach, H.I., Eds. 1995. *Irritant Dermatitis Syndrome,* CRC Press, Boca Raton, FL.

REFERENCES

1. Weltfriend, S., Bason, M., Lammintausta, K., Maibach, H.I., Irritant dermatitis (irritation). In: Marzulli, F., Maibach, H., Eds., *Dermatoxicology.* Washinton, D.C.: Taylor & Francis, 1995:87–118.
2. Elsner, P., Berardesca, E., Maibach, H., *Bioengineering of the Skin: Water and the Stratum Corneum.* Boca Raton, FL: CRC Press, 1994.
3. van der Valk, P.G.M., Maibach, H.I., *Irritant Dermatitis Syndrome.* Boca Raton, FL: CRC Press, 1995.
4. Fregert, S.F., Irritant contact dermatitis. In Fregert, S.F., Ed., *Manual of Contact Dermatitis.* Copenhagen: Munksgaard, 1981:55–62.
5. Griffiths, W.A.D., Wilkinson, D.S., Primary irritants and solvents. In Griffiths, W.A.D., Wilkinson, D.S., Eds., *Essentials of Industrial Dermatology.* Oxford: Blackwell Scientific, 1985:58–72.
6. Hjorth, N., Avnstorp, C., Rehabilitation in hand eczema. *Derm. Beruf. Umwelt.* 1986; 34:74–76.

7. Malten, K.E., den Arend, J.A., Wiggers, R.E., Delayed irritation: hexanediol diacrylate and butanediol diacrylate. *Contact Dermatitis* 1979; 5:178–184.

8. Lovell, C.R., Rycroft, R.J., Williams, D.M., Hamlin, J.W., Contact dermatitis from the irritancy (immediate and delayed) and allergenicity of hydroxypropyl acrylate. *Contact Dermatitis* 1985; 12:117–118.

9. Malten, K.E., den Arend, J., Topical toxicity of various concentrations of DMSO recorded with impedance measurements and water vapour loss measurements: recording of skin's adaptation to repeated DMSO irritation. *Contact Dermatitis* 1978; 4:80–92.

10. von Hagerman, G., Uber das "traumaterative" (toxische) Ekzem. *Dermatologica* 1957; 115:525–529.

11. Agrup, G., Hand eczema and other dermatoses in South Sweden (Thesis.). *Acta Derm. Venereol.* (Suppl.) 1969; 49:61.

12. Marrakchi, S., Maibach, H.I., What is occupational contact dermatitis? An operational definition. *Dermatol. Clin.* 1994; 12:477–484.

13. Ale, S.I., Maibach, H.I., Clinical relevance in allergic contact dermatitis. An algorithmic approach. *Derm. Beruf. Umwelt.* 1995; 43:119–121.

14. Maibach, H.I., Mathias, C.T., Vulvar dermatitis and fissures — irritant dermatitis from methyl benzethonium chloride. *Contact Dermatitis* 1985; 13:340.

15. Wahlberg, J.E., Maibach, H.I., Identification of contact pustulogens. In Marzulli FN, Maibach HI, Eds., *Dermatotoxicology*. New York: Hemisphere, 1982:627–635.

16. Dooms-Goossens, E., Debusschere, K.M., Gevers, D.M. et al., Contact dermatitis caused by airborne agents. A review and case reports. *J. Am. Acad. Dermatol.* 1986; 15:1–10.

17. Fischer, T., Rystedt, I., False-positive, follicular and irritant patch test reactions to metal salts. *Contact Dermatitis* 1985; 12:93–98.

18. Wahlberg, JE.,. Maibach, H.I., Sterile cutaneous pustules: a manifestation of primary irritancy? Identification of contact pustulogens. *J. Invest. Dermatol.* 1981; 76:381–383.

19. Berardesca, E., Maibach, H.I., Racial differences in sodium lauryl sulphate induced cutaneous irritation: black and white. *Contact Dermatitis* 1988; 18:65–70.

20. van der Valk, P.G., Nater, J.P., Bleumink, E., Vulnerability of the skin to surfactants in different groups of eczema patients and controls as measured by water vapour loss. *Clin. Exp. Dermatol.* 1985; 10:98–103.

21. Lammintausta, K., Maibach, H.I., Wilson, D., Mechanisms of subjective (sensory) irritation. Propensity to non-immunologic contact urticaria and objective irritation in stingers. *Derm. Beruf. Umwelt.* 1988; 36:45–49.

22. Frosch, P., Kligman, A., Recognition of chemically vulnerable and delicate skin. In *Principles of Cosmetics for Dermatologists*. St. Louis: C.V. Mosby, 1982:287–296.

23. Lahti, A., Maibach, H., Guinea pig ear swelling as an animal model for nonimmunologic contact urticaria. In Maibach, H., Lowe, N., Eds., *Models in Dermatology*. Vol. II. New York: S. Karger, 1985:356–359.

24. Berardesca, E., Cespa, M., Farinelli, N., Rabbiosi, G., Maibach, H., *In vivo* transcutaneous penetration of nicotinates and sensitive skin. *Contact Dermatitis* 1991; 25:35–38.

25. Cua, A.B., Wilhelm, K.P., Maibach, H.I., Skin surface lipid and skin friction: relation to age, sex and anatomical region. *Skin Pharmacol.* 1995; 8:246–251.

26. Kligman, A.M., Wooding, W.M., A method for the measurement and evaluation of irritants on human skin. *J. Invest. Dermatol.* 1967; 49:78–94.

27. Nangia, A., Bloom, E., Berner, B., Maibach, H.I., Influence of skin irritants on percutaneous absorption. *Pharm. Res.,* 1993; 10:1756–1759.

28. Rothenborg, H.W., Menne, T., Sjolin, K.E., Temperature dependent primary irritant dermatitis from lemon perfume. *Contact Dermatitis* 1977; 3:37–48.
29. Cooper, E., Vehicle effects on skin penetration. In Maibach, H., Bronaugh, R., Eds., *Percutaneous Absorption*. New York: Marcel Dekker, 1985:525–530.
30. Gummer, C., Vehicles as penetration enhancers. In Maibach H, Bronaugh R, Eds., *Percutaneous Absorption*. New York: Marcel Dekker, 1985:561–570.
31. Smith, E., Maibach, H.I., *Percutaneous Penetration Enhancers*. Boca Raton, FL: CRC Press, 1995.
32. Maibach, H.I., Dermatologic vehicles. Science and art. *Cutis* 1995; 55:4–16.
33. Flannigan, S.A., Tucker, S.B., Influence of the vehicle on irritant contact dermatitis. *Contact Dermatitis* 1985; 12:177–178.
34. Lammintausta, K., Maibach, H.I., Wilson, D., Susceptibility to cumulative and acute irritant dermatitis. An experimental approach in human volunteers. *Contact Dermatitis* 1988; 19:84–90.
35. Malten, K.E., Thoughts on irritant contact dermatitis. *Contact Dermatitis* 1981; 7:238–247.
36. Patil, S.M., Singh, P., Maibach, H.I., Cumulative irritancy to sodium lauryl sulfate: The overlap phenomenon. *Int. J. Pharm.* 1994; 110:147–154.
37. Patil, S.M., Singh, P., Maibach, H.I., Quantification of sodium lauryl sulfate (SLS) penetration into the skin and underlying tissues after topical applicaton — pharmacological and toxicological implications. *J. Pharm. Sci.* 1995; 84:1240–1244.
38. Patil, S.M., Singh, P., Maibach, H.I., Radial spread of sodium lauryl sulfate below a topical application. *Pharm. Res.* 1995; 12:2018–2023.
39. Lammintausta, K., Maibach, H.I., Wilson, D., Human cutaneous irritation: induced hyporeactivity. *Contact Dermatitis* 1987; 17:193–198.
40. Pittz, E., Smorbeck, R., Rieger, M., An animal test procedure for the simultaneous assessment of irritancy and efficacy of skin care products. In Maibach, H., Lowe, N., Eds., *Models in Dermatology*. Vol. II. New York: S. Karger, 1985:209–224.
41. Susten, A.S., The chronic effects of mechanical trauma to the skin: a review of the literature. *Am. J. Ind. Med.* 1985; 8:281–288.
42. Hannuksela, M., Pirila, V., Salo, O.P., Skin reactions to propylene glycol. *Contact Dermatitis* 1975; 1:112–116.
43. Rycroft, R.J., Occupational dermatoses from warm dry air. *Br. J. Dermatol.* 1981; 105 Suppl 21:29–34.
44. Agner, T., Serup, J., Seasonal variation of skin resistance to irritants. *Br. J. Dermatol.* 1989; 121:323–8.
45. van der Valk, P.G., Maibach, H.I., Post-application occlusion substantially increases the irritant response of the skin to repeated short-term sodium lauryl sulfate (SLS) exposure. *Contact Dermatitis* 1989; 21:335–338.
46. Jambor, J.J., Etiologic appraisal of hand dermatitis. *J. Invest. Dermatol.* 1955; 24:387–392.
47. Bettley, F.R., Some effects of soap on the skin. *Br. Med. J.* 1960; 1:1675–1679.
48. Suskind, R.R., Meister, M.M., Scheen, S.R. et al., Cutaneous effects of household synthetic detergents and soaps. *Arch. Dermatol.* 1963; 88:117–124.
49. Stoughton, R.B., Potts, L.W., Clendenning, W. et al., Management of patients with eczematous diseases: use of soap vs. no soap. *JAMA* 1969; 175:1196–1198.
50. White, M.I., Jenkinson, D.M., Lloyd, D.H., The effect of washing on the thickness of the stratum corneum in normal and atopic individuals. *Br. J. Dermatol.* 1987; 116:525–530.

51. Bjornberg, A., Skin reactions to primary irritants in patients with hand eczema. Oscar Isacsons Tryckeri AB, Gothenburg, Sweden, 1968.

52. Thiele, F.A., Malten, K.E., Evaluation of skin damage. I. Skin resistance measurements with alternating current (impedance measurements). *Br. J. Dermatol.* 1973; 89:373–382.

53. Maibach, H., Bronaugh, R., Guy, R., Noninvasive techniques for determining skin function. In Drill, V., Lazar, P., Eds., *Cutaneous Toxicity*. New York: Raven Press, 1984:63–97.

54. Tagami, H., Ohi, M., Iwatsuki, K., Kanamaru, Y., Yamada, M., Ichijo, B., Evaluation of the skin surface hydration *in vivo* by electrical measurement. *J. Invest. Dermatol.* 1980; 75:500–507.

55. Guy, R.H., Tur, E., Maibach, H.I., Optical techniques for monitoring cutaneous microcirculation. Recent applications. *Int. J. Dermatol.* 1985; 24:88–94.

56. Maibach, H.I., Feldman, R.J., Milby, T.H., Serat, W.F., Regional variation in percutaneous penetration in man. Pesticides. *Arch. Environ. Health* 1971; 23:208–211.

57. Grice, K., Sattar, H., Baker, H., Epstein, E., The cutaneous barrier to salts and water in psoriasis and in normal skin. Contact dermatitis in children. *Br. J. Dermatol.* 1973; 88:459–463.

58. Frame, G.W., Strauss, W.G., Maibach, H.I., Carbon dioxide emission of the human arm and hand. *J. Invest. Dermatol.* 1972; 59:155–159.

59. Grice, K., Sattar, H., Casey, T., Baker, H., An evaluation of Na^+, Cl^- and pH ion-specific electrodes in the study of the electrolyte contents of epidermal transudate and sweat. *Br. J. Dermatol.* 1975; 92:511–518.

60. Berardesca, E., Elsner, P., Maibach, H., *Bioengineering of the Skin, Cutaneous Blood Flow and Erythema*. Boca Raton, FL: CRC Press, 1994.

61. Serup, J., Jemec, G.B.E., Noninvasive techniques for assessments of skin penetration and bioavailability. *Handbook of Non-Invasive Methods and the Skin*. Boca Raton, FL: CRC Press, 1995:201–205.

62. Elsner, P., Berardesca, E., Wilhelm, K., Maibach, H.I., *Bioengineering of the Skin: Methods and Instrumentation*. Boca Raton, FL: CRC Press, 1995.

63. Ummenhofer, B., [On the method for testing alkali resistance (author's transl)]. *Derm. Beruf. Umwelt.* 1980; 28:104–109.

64. Wilhelm, K.P., Pasche, F., Surber, C., Maibach, H.I., Sodium hydroxide-induced subclinical irritation. A test for evaluating stratum corneum barrier function. *Acta Derm. Venereol.* 1990; 70:463–467.

65. Frosch, P.J., *Hautirritation und Empfindliche Haut*. Berlin: Grosse Verlag, 1985:1–118.

66. Lee, C.H., Maibach, H.I., SLS — an overview. *Contact Dermatitis* 1995; 33:1–7.

67. Feldmann, R.J., Maibach, H.I., Regional variation in percutaneous penetration of 14C cortisol in man. *J. Invest. Dermatol.* 1967; 48:181–183.

68. Cronin, E., Stoughton, R.B.L., Percutaneous absorption: regional variation and the effect of hydration and epidermal stripping. *Br. J. Dermatol.* 1962; 74:7265–7272.

69. Wester, R.C., Maibach, H.I., Dermatopharmacokinetics. In Maibach, H.I., Bronaugh, R.L., Eds., *Clinical Dermatology in Percutaneous Absorption*. New York: Marcel Dekker, 1985:525–530.

70. Wester, R., Maibach, H., Regional variation in percutaneous absorption. In Bronaugh, R., Maibach, H.I., Eds., New York: Marcel Dekker, 1989:111–119.

71. Tur, E., Maibach, H.I., Guy, R.H., Spatial variability of vasodilatation in human forearm skin. *Br. J. Dermatol.* 1985; 113:197–203.

72. Magnusson, B., Hersle, K., Patch test methods: II. Regional variation of patch test responses. *Acta Derm. Venereol.* 1965; 45:226–257.
73. Flannigan, S.A., Smith, R.E., McGovern, J.P., Intraregional variation between contact irritant patch test sites. *Contact Dermatitis* 1984; 10:123–124.
74. Hornstein, O.P., Kienlein-Kletschka, B.M., Improvement of patch test allergen exposure by short-term local pressure. *Dermatologica* 1982; 165:607–611.
75. Gollhausen, R., Kligman, A.M., Effects of pressure on contact dermatitis. *Am. J. Ind. Med.* 1985; 8:223–228.
76. Britz, M.B., Maibach, H.I., Human cutaneous vulvar reactivity to irritants. *Contact Dermatitis* 1979; 5:375–377.
77. Oriba, H.A., Elsner, P., Maibach, H.I., Vulvar physiology. *Semin. Dermatol.* 1989; 8:2–6.
78. Jordan, W., Blaney, T., Factors influencing infant diaper dermatitis. In Maibach, H., Boisits, E., Eds., *Neonatal Skin: Structure and Function.* New York: Marcel Dekker, 1982:205–221.
79. Barrett, D., Rutter, N., Transdermal delivery and the premature neonate. *Crit. Rev. Ther. Drug Carrier Syst.* 1994; 11:1–30.
80. Seymour, J.L., Keswick, B.H., Hanifin, J.M., Jordan, W.P., Milligan, M.C., Clinical effects of diaper types on the skin of normal infants and infants with atopic dermatitis. *J. Am. Acad. Dermatol.* 1987; 17:988–997.
81. Mobly, S.L., Mansmann, H.C., Current status of skin testing in children with contact dermatitis. *Cutis* 1974; 13:995–1000.
82. Epstein, E., Contact dermatitis in children. *Pediatr. Clin. North Am.* 1971; 18:839–852.
83. Fisher, A.A., Childhood allergic contact dermatitis. *Cutis* 1975; 15:635–642.
84. Maibach, H., Boisits, E., Neonatal skin: structure and function. New York: Marcel Dekker, 1982.
85. Beauregard, S., Gilchrest, B.A., A survey of skin problems and skin care regimens in the elderly. *Arch. Dermatol.* 1987; 123:1638–1643.
86. Lejman, E., Stoudemayer, T., Grove, G., Kligman, A.M., Age differences in poison ivy dermatitis. *Contact Dermatitis* 1984; 11:163–167.
87. Grove, G.L., Lavker, R.M., Hoelzle, E. et al., Use of nonintrusive tests to monitor age-associated changes in human skin. *J. Soc. Cosmet. Chem.* 1981; 32:15–26.
88. Frosch, P.J., Kligman, A.M., Rapid blister formation in human skin with ammonium hydroxide. *Br. J. Dermatol.* 1977; 96:461–473.
89. Kligman, A.M., Perspectives and problems in cutaneous gerontology. *J. Invest. Dermatol.* 1979; 73:39–46.
90. Roskos, K.V., Maibach, H.I., Percutaneous absorption and age. Implications for therapy. *Drugs Aging* 1992; 2:432–449.
91. Christophers, E., Kligman, A., Percutaneous absorption in aged skin. In Montagna, E., Ed., *Advances in the Biology of the Skin.* Oxford: Pergamon Press, 1965:160–179.
92. Tagami, H., Functional characteristics of aged skin. *Acta Derm. Venereol.* 1971; 66:19–21.
93. DeSalva, S.J., Thompson, G., ^{22}NaCl skin clearance in humans and its relation to skin age. *J. Invest. Dermatol.* 1965; 45:315–318.
94. Guy, R.H., Tur, E., Bjerke, S., Maibach, H.I., Are there age and racial differences to methyl nicotinate-induced vasodilatation in human skin? *J. Am. Acad. Dermatol.* 1985; 12:1001–1006.
95. Kwangsukstith, C., Maibach, H.I., Effect of age and sex on irritant and allergic contact dermatitis. *Contact Dermatitis* 1995; 33:289–298.

96. Elias, P.M., Lipids and the epidermal permeability barrier. *Arch. Dermatol. Res.* 1981; 270:95–117.

97. Gilchrest, B.A., Murphy, G.F., Soter, N.A., Effect of chronologic aging and ultraviolet irradiation on Langerhans cells in human epidermis. *J. Invest. Dermatol.* 1982; 79:85–88.

98. Roberts, D., Marks, R., The determination of regional and age variations in the rate of desquamation: a comparison of four techniques. *J. Invest. Dermatol.* 1980; 74:13–16.

99. Baker, H., Blair, C.P., Cell replacement in the human stratum corenum in old age. *Br. J. Dermatol.* 1968; 80:367–372.

100. Montagna, W., Carlisle, K., Structural changes in aging human skin. *J. Invest. Dermatol.* 1979; 73:47–53.

101. Holzle, E., Plewig, G., Ledolter, A., Corneocyte exfoliative cytology: A model to study normal and diseased stratum corneum. In Marks, R., Plewig, G., Eds., *Skin Models*. New York: Springer Verlag, 1986:183–193.

102. Weigand, D.A., Gaylor, J.R., Irritant reaction in Negro and Caucasian skin. *South Med. J.* 1974; 67:548–551.

103. Andersen, K.E., Maibach, H.I., Black and white human skin differences. *J. Am. Acad. Dermatol.* 1979; 1:276–282.

104. Johnson, L.C., Corah, N.L., Racial skin differences in skin resistance. *Science* 1960; 139:766–767.

105. Weigand, D.A., Haygood, C., Gaylor, J.R., Cell layers and density of Negro and Caucasian stratum corneum. *J. Invest. Dermatol.* 1974; 62:563–568.

106. Buckley, C., Lee, K.L., Burdick, D.S., Methacholine-induced cutaneous flare response: bivariate analysis of responsiveness and sensitivity. *J. Allergy Clin. Immunol.* 1982; 69:25–34.

107. Buckley, C., Larrick, J.W., Kaplan, J.E., Population differences in cutaneous methacholine reactivity and circulating IgE concentrations. *J. Allergy Clin. Immunol.* 1985; 76:847–854.

108. Berardesca, E., Maibach, H.I., Racial differences in skin pathophysiology. *J. Am. Acad. Dermatol.* 1996; 34:667–672.

109. Rystedt, I., Factors influencing the occurrence of hand eczema in adults with a history of atopic dermatitis in childhood. *Contact Dermatitis* 1985; 12:185–191.

110. Lantingna, H., Nater, J.P., Coenraads, P.J., Prevalence, incidence and course of eczema on the hands and forearms in a sample of the general population. *Contact Dermatitis* 1984; 10:135–139.

111. Wagner, G., Porschel, W., Klinisch-analytische Studie zum Neurodermatitisproblem. *Dermatologica* 1962; 125:1–32.

112. Magnusson, B., Hillgren, L., Skin irritating and adhesive characteristics of some different adhesive tapes. *Acta Derm. Venereol.* 1962; 42:463–472.

113. Bjornberg, A., Skin reactions to primary irritants in men and women. *Acta Derm. Venereol.* 1975; 55:191–194.

114. Lammintausta, K., Maibach, H.I., Wilson, D., Irritant reactivity in males and females. *Contact Dermatitis* 1987; 17:276–280.

115. Olumide, Y., Contact dermatitis in Nigeria. (II). Hand dermatitis in men. *Contact Dermatitis* 1987; 17:136–138.

116. Holst, R., Moller, H., One hundred twin pairs patch tested with primary irritants. *Br. J. Dermatol.* 1975; 93:145–149.

117. Frosch, P.J., Wissing, C., Cutaneous sensitivity to ultraviolet light and chemical irritants. *Arch. Dermatol. Res.* 1982; 272:269–278.

118. Maurice, P.D., Greaves, M.W., Relationship between skin type and erythemal response to anthralin. *Br. J. Dermatol.* 1983; 109:337–341.
119. Czerwinska-Dihm, I., Rudzki, E., Skin reactions to primary irritants. *Contact Dermatitis* 1981; 7:315–319.
120. Hanifin, J.M., Rajka, G., Diagnostic features of atopic dermatitis. *Acta Derm. Venereol.* 1980; Suppl. 92:44–47.
121. Ziierz, P., Kiessling, W., Berg, A., Experimentelle Prufung der Hautfunktion bei Icthyosis Vulgaris. *Arch. Klin. Exp. Dermatol.* 1960; 209:592.
122. Hanifin, J.M., Lobitz, W.C., Jr., Newer concepts of atopic dermatitis. *Arch. Dermatol.* 1977; 113:663–670.
123. Skog, E., Primary irritant and allergic eczematous reactions in patients with different dermatoses. *Acta Derm. Venereol.* 1960; 40:307.
124. Rajka, G., The aetiology of atopic dermatitis. In Rajka, G., Ed., *Atopic Dermatitis.* Philadelphia: W.B. Saunders, 1975:46–104.
125. Werner, Y., Lindberg, M., Forslind, B., The water-binding capacity of stratum corneum in dry non-eczematous skin of atopic eczema. *Acta Derm. Venereol.* 1982; 62:334–337.
126. Finlay, A.Y., Nicholls, S., King, C.S., Marks, R., The "dry" non-eczematous skin associated with atopic eczema. *Br. J. Dermatol.* 1980; 103:249–256.
127. Al-Jaberi, H., Marks, R., Studies of the clinically uninvolved skin in patients with dermatitis. *Br. J. Dermatol.* 1984; 111:437–443.
128. Gloor, M., Heymann, B., Stuhlert, T., Infrared-spectroscopic determination of the water content of the horny layer in healthy subjects and in patients suffering from atopic dermatitis. *Arch. Dermatol. Res.* 1981; 271:429–436.
129. Lammintausta, K., Kalimo, K., Atopy and hand dermatitis in hospital wet work. *Contact Dermatitis* 1981; 7:301–308.
130. Vickers, H.R., The influence of age on the onset of dermatitis in industry. Paper presented at Symposium Dermatologorum de Morbis Cutaneis, Prague, 1962.
131. Holland, B.D., Occupational dermatoses — predisposing and direct causes. *JAMA* 1958; 167:2203–2205.
132. Hornstein, O.P., Baurle, G., Kienlein-Kletschka, B., [Prospective study of the importance of constitutional parameters in the development of eczema in hairdressers and construction workers]. *Derm. Beruf. Umwelt.* 1985; 33:43–49.
133. Kingston, T., Marks, R., Irritant reactions to dithranol in normal subjects and psoriatic patients. *Br. J. Dermatol.* 1983; 108:307–313.
134. Lawrence, C.M., Howel, D., Shuster, S., The inflammatory response to anthralin. *Clin. Exp. Dermatol.* 1984; 9:336–341.
135. MacDonald, K.J., Marks, J., Short contact anthralin in the treatment of psoriasis: a study of different contact times. *Br. J. Dermatol.* 1986; 114:235–239.
136. Epstein, E., Maibach, H.I., Eczematous psoriasis: what is it? In Roenigk, H.H., Jr., Maibach, H.I., Eds., *Psoriasis.* New York: Marcel Dekker, 1985:9–14.
137. Mitchell, J.C., Angry back syndrome [letter]. *Contact Dermatitis* 1981; 7:359–361.
138. Bruynzeel, D.P., van Ketel, W.G., von Blomberg-van der Flier, M., Scheper, R.J., Angry back or the excited skin syndrome. A prospective study. *J. Am. Acad. Dermatol.* 1983; 8:392–397.
139. Bruynzeel, D.P., Maibach, H.I., Excited skin syndrome (angry back). *Arch. Dermatol.* 1986; 122:323–328.
140. Nilsson, E., Mikaelsson, B., Andersson, S., Atopy, occupation and domestic work as risk factors for hand eczema in hospital workers. *Contact Dermatitis* 1985; 13:216–223.

141. Johansen, J.D., Ramsing, D., Vejlsgaard, G., Agner, T., Skin barrier properties in patients with recessive X-linked icthyosis. *Acta Derm. Venereol.* 1995; 75:202–204.
142. van der Valk, P.G., Nater, J.P., Bleumink, E., Skin irritancy of surfactants as assessed by water vapor loss measurements. *J. Invest. Dermatol.* 1984; 82:291–293.
143. Elsner, P., Maibach, H., Irritant dermatitis syndrome. New York, S. Karger, 1995.
144. Blanken, R., van der Valk, P.G., Nater, J.P., Laser-Doppler flowmetry in the investigation of irritant compounds on human skin. *Derm. Beruf. Umwelt.* 1986; 34:5–9.
145. Pinnagoda, J., Tupker, R.A., Agner, T., Serup, J., Guidelines for transepidermal water loss (TEWL) measurement. A report from the Standardization Group of the European Society of *Contact Dermatitis. Contact Dermatitis* 1990; 22:164–178.
146. Csato, M., Czarnetzki, B.M., Effect of BN 52021, a platelet activating factor antagonist, on experimental murine contact dermatitis. *Br. J. Dermatol.* 1988; 118:475–479.
147. Rosenbach, T., Csato, M., Czarnetzki, B.M., Studies on the role of leukotrienes in murine allergic and irritant contact dermatitis. *Br. J. Dermatol.* 1988; 118:1–6.
148. Frosch, P.J., Czarnetzki, B.M., Surfactants cause *in vitro* chemotaxis and chemokinesis of human neutrophils. *J. Invest. Dermatol.* 1987:52s–55s.
149. Gawkrodger, D.J., Carr, M.M., McVittie, E., Guy, K., Hunter, J.A., Keratinocyte expression of MHC class II antigens in allergic sensitization and challenge reactions and in irritant contact dermatitis. *J. Invest. Dermatol.* 1987; 88:11–16.
150. Johnson, M.W., Maibach, H.I., Salmon, S.E., Skin reactivity in patients with cancer. Impaired delayed hypersensitivity or faulty inflammatory response? *N. Engl. J. Med.* 1971; 284:1255–1257.
151. Weidenfeld, S., Beitrage zur Pathogenese des Ekzems. *Arch. Dermatol. Syphilol.* 1912; 13:891.
152. Schultz, I.H., Beitrag zum klinischen Studium und der quantatitiven Pruefung der Hautreaktion auf chemische Reize. I. Mitteilung: Uber das Verhalten normaler und leukopathischer Hautstellen Hautkranker und Hautreaktion bei peripheren und zentraelen Lahmungen. *Arch. Dermatol. Syphilol.* 1912; 13:987.
153. Halter, K., Zur Pathogenese des Ekzems. *Arch. Dermatol. Syphilol.* 1941; 181:593.
154. Bjornberg, A., Feuerman, E., Levy, A., Skin reactions to primary irritants and predisposition to eczema. A study of the effect of prednisone and an antihistamine on patch test reactions. *Br. J. Dermatol.* 1974; 91:425–427.
155. Biberstein, H., The effects of unilateral cervical sympathectomy on reactions of the skin. *J. Invest. Dermatol.* 1940; 3:201.
156. Schaefer, W., Beitrag zum kinischen Studium und der quantatitiven Pruefung der Hautreaktion auf chemische Reize. II. Uber die chemische Hautreaktion bei peripheren und zentralen Lahmungen. *Arch. Dermatol. Syphilol.* 1921; 132:87.
157. Kaufman, A.M., Winkel, M., Entzuendung und Nervensystem. *Klin. Wochenschr.* 1922; 1:12.
158. Foster, R.W., Ramage, A.G., Evidence for a specific somatosensory receptor in the cat skin that responds to irritant chemicals [proceedings]. *Br. J. Pharmacol.* 1976; 57:436P.
159. Nilzen, A., Wikstrom, K., Factors influencing the skin reaction in guinea pigs sensitized with 2,4-dinitrochlorobenzene. *Acta Derm. Venereol.* 1955; 35:415.
160. Goldman, L., Preston, R., Rockwell, E., The local effect of 17-hydroxycorticosterone-21-acetate (compound F) on the diagnostic patch test reaction. *J. Invest. Dermatol.* 1952; 18:89.
161. Feuerman, E., Maibach, H.I., A study of the effect of prednisone and an antihistamine on patch test reactions. *Br. J. Dermatol.* 1972; 86:68.
162. Funk, J.O., Maibach, H.I., Horizons in pharmacologic intervention in allergic contact dermatitis. *J. Am. Acad. Dermatol.* 1994; 31:999–1014.

163. Phillips, L., Steinberg, M., Maibach, H.I., Akers, W.A., A comparison of rabbit and human skin response to certain irritants. *Toxicol. Appl. Pharmacol.* 1972; 21:369–382.

164. National Research Council, Principles and procedures for evaluating the toxicity of household substances. National Academy of Sciences, Washington, D.C., 1977.

165. Marzulli, F.N., Maibach, H.I., The rabbit as a model for evaluating skin irritants: a comparison of results obtained on animals and man using repeated skin exposures. *Food Cosmet. Toxicol.* 1975; 13:533–540.

166. Steinberg, M., Akers, W., Weeks, M., McCreesh, A., Maibach, H., A comparison of test techniques based on rabbit and human skin responses to irritants with recommendations regarding the evaluation of mildly or moderately irritating compounds. In Maibach, H., Ed., *Animal Models in Dermatology*. New York: Churchill Livingstone, 1975:1–11.

167. Frosch, P., Kligman, A., The chamber scarification test for assessing irritancy of topically applied substances. In Drill, V., Lazar, P., Eds., *Cutaneous Toxicity*. New York: Academic Press, 1977:150.

168. Rollins, T.G., From xerosis to nummular dermatitis: The dehydration dermatoses. *JAMA* 1978; 206:637.

169. Spruit, D., Evaluation of skin function by the alkali application technique. *Curr. Probl. Dermatol.* 1970; 3:148.

170. Spruit, D., Interference of some substances with vapor loss of human skin. *Am. Perfum. Cosmet.* 1971; 8:27.

171. Malten, K.E., Thiele, F.A., Evaluation of skin damage. II. Water loss and carbon dioxide release measurements related to skin resistance measurements. *Br. J. Dermatol.* 1973; 89:565–569.

172. Thiele, F.A.J., *Measurements on the Surface of the Skin*. Nijmegen, Netherlands: Drukkeij van Mammeren BV, 1974:81.

173. Anjo. D.M., Cunico, R.L., Maibach, H.I., Transepidermal chloride diffusion in man. *Clin. Res.* 1978; 26:208A.

174. Lo, J.S., Oriba, H.A., Maibach, H.I., Bailin, P.L., Transepidermal potassium ion, chloride ion, and water flux across delipidized and cellophane tape-stripped skin. *Dermatologica* 1990; 180:66–68.

175. Gross, P., Blade, M.O., Chester, J., Sloane, M.B., Dermatitis of housewives as a variation of nummular eczema. A study of pH of the skin and alkali neutralization by the Burckhart technique. Further advances in therapy and prophylaxis. *Arch. Dermatol.* 1954; 70:94.

176. Frosch, P.J., Rapid blister formation in human skin with ammonium hydroxide, Society of Investigative Dermatology, San Francisco, CA, 1978.

177. Rougier, A., Goldberg, A.M., Maibach, H.I., *In Vitro Skin Toxicology: Irritation, Phototoxicity, Sensitization*. (Alternative Methods in Toxicology Series, Vol. 10.) New York: Mary Ann Liebert, Inc., 1994.

178. Scheynius, A., Fischer, T., Forsum, U., Klareskog, L., Phenotypic characterization *in situ* of inflammatory cells in allergic and irritant contact dermatitis in man. *Clin. Exp. Immunol.* 1984; 55:81–90.

179. Ferguson, J., Gibbs, J.H., Beck, J.S., Lymphocyte subsets and Langerhans cells in allergic and irritant patch test reactions: histometric studies. *Contact Dermatitis* 1985; 13:166–174.

180. Avnstorp, C., Ralfkiaer, E., Jorgensen, J., Wantzin, G.L., Sequential immunophenotypic study of lymphoid infiltrate in allergic and irritant reactions. *Contact Dermatitis* 1987; 16:239–245.

181. Anderson, K.E., Sjolin, K.E., Soelgaard, P., Acute irritant contact folliculitis in a galvanizer, paper presented at European Symposium on *Contact Dermatitis*, Heidelberg, 1988.

182. Patrick, E., Burkhalter, A., Maibach, H.I., Recent investigations of mechanisms of chemically induced skin irritation in laboratory mice. *J. Invest. Dermatol.* 1987:24s–31s.

183. Ruzicka, T., Printz, M.P., Arachidonic acid metabolism in skin: experimental contact dermatitis in guinea pigs. *Int. Arch. Allerg. Appl. Immunol.* 1982; 69:347–352.

184. Epstein, W., Cutaneous granulomas as a toxicologic problem. In Marzulli, F., Maibach, H., Eds., *Dermatoxicology*. New York: Hemisphere Publishing, 1983:533–545.

185. Kresbach, H., Kerl, H., Wawschinek, O., [Mercury granuloma of the skin]. *Berufsdermatosen* 1971; 19:173–186.

186. Andres, T.L., Vallyathan, N.V., Madison, J.F., Electron-probe microanalysis. Aid in the study of skin granulomas. *Arch. Dermatol.* 1980; 116:1272–1274.

187. McOsker, D.E., Beck, L.W., Characteristics of accommodated (hardened) skin. *J. Invest. Dermatol.* 1967; 48:372–383.

188. Thorvaldsen, J., Volden, G., PUVA-induced diminution of contact allergic and irritant skin reactions. *Clin. Exp. Dermatol.* 1980; 5:43–46.

189. Camel, E., O'Connell, M., Gross, M., Sage, B., Maibach, H.I., Iontophoresis: Irritation I. *Fund. Appl. Toxicol.* 1996; 32:168–178.

190. Camel, E., Gross, M., Sage, B., Maibach, H.I., Iontopheresis: Irritation II. (to be submitted for publication).

191. Feldmann, R.J., Maibach, H.I., Systemic absorption of pesticides through the skin of man. Occupational exposure to pesticides. Report to the Federal Working Group on pest management from the Task Group on Occupational Exposure to Pesticides, Appendix B, pp. 120–127, 1974.

5 Pharmacokinetics and Dynamics of Temporal Delivery

Ronald R. Burnette

CONTENTS

5.1   INTRODUCTION

The parameters governing the pharmacokinetics and the pharmacodynamics of a drug do not necessarily remain constant. In fact, many of these parameters undergo circadian (24-h period) rhythms.[1-5] These periodic alterations in parameter values can result in a periodic modulation of plasma drug levels and drug effects even if the drug is infused at a constant rate intravenously to steady state. In addition, a patient's tolerance to drugs and the patient's disease status can vary in a circadian manner. Based on this, it would seem reasonable that one might be able to achieve, by the proper modulation of drug delivery, a maximum therapeutic effect while at the same time producing minimal toxicity. An excellent discussion of several aspects of the pharmacokinetics and dynamics of temporal drug delivery has already been provided by Levy.[4] In his paper, he outlines qualitatively the main factors one should consider in the design of temporal drug delivery systems. In this chapter, the intent will be to extend these ideas in a more quantitative sense. In particular, simulations (based on experimental data) will be used to demonstrate the influence that circadian rhythms and modulated drug delivery have on a patient's therapeutic and toxic response to a drug. This will be done in conjunction with a conceptual framework, based on physical and physiological insight, which can be used to explain the observed results.

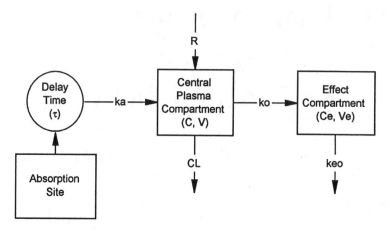

FIGURE 5.1 A model describing the temporal delivery of drug in the body. The body is treated as one central compartment having a plasma concentration of C, an apparent plasma volume of distribution of V, a clearance of CL, and an input infusion rate of R which can be a function of time. The effect compartment is connected to the central plasma compartment through a mass transfer rate constant of ko. The effect compartment has a concentration of Ce, a volume Ve, and an elimination rate constant of keo. Drugs that are administered extravascularly are given at the absorption site. The delay time between the absorption site and the central compartment is given by τ and the absorption rate constant connecting the absorption site to the central compartment is ka.

5.2   DESCRIPTION OF THE MODEL

The model will consist of an absorption compartment, a central plasma compartment having a plasma concentration of C, and an effect compartment having an effect concentration equal to Ce (Figure 5.1). To aid in more clearly delineating the factors influencing this model, we will focus on only portions of this model rather than the model in its entirety. The central plasma compartment will have a plasma clearance (CL) and an apparent plasma volume of distribution (V) yielding an elimination rate constant equal to the clearance divided by the volume of distribution. The absorption compartment will be connected to the central plasma compartment, through a delay time (τ), by a mass transfer coefficient equal to ka. Modulation of the CL, V, and ka is allowed. The effect compartment is connected to the central plasma compartment by a mass transfer rate coefficient ko. The effect compartment will also have a first-order elimination rate coefficient keo. The mass transfer from the central plasma compartment into the effect compartment can be assumed to be approximately zero. Finally, the effect will be assumed to be receptor mediated and that the response of the receptor can be modulated. Modulation of drug delivery will initially be assumed to occur as a pure sinusoidally varying input which will have a period of 24 h. This type of temporal delivery profile was chosen because most factors influencing the pharmacokinetics, pharmacodynamics, toxicity, and disease status also have oscillation periods of approximately 24 h. Thus, the basic approach taken will be to show how, by properly adjusting the phase shifts (time lags) between the temporal drug delivery system and the body's inherent circadian rhythms, one can maximize therapeutic efficacy.

5.3 THEORETICAL DESCRIPTION OF SPECIAL CASES OF THE MODEL

Figure 5.1 can be used to determine the mass balance equations used in obtaining the results given in Figures 5.2 through 5.7. In Figure 5.2, just the central plasma compartment is considered under conditions where the rate of infusion is either constant or modulated. Thus, we have for a constant rate of infusion directly into the central compartment

$$\frac{dC}{dt} = -\left(\frac{CL}{V}\right) \cdot C + \frac{Ro}{V} \tag{5.1}$$

where Ro is the constant rate of infusion. If the rate of infusion is now modulated, we have

$$\frac{dC}{dt} = -\left(\frac{CL}{V}\right) \cdot C + \frac{Ro \cdot \left(1 + \sin\left(\frac{2 \cdot \pi \, t}{tp}\right)\right)}{V} \tag{5.2}$$

where t is time and tp is the period of the sine wave.

In Figure 5.3, which allows for either a constant or a modulated drug clearance, the central compartment concentration is described by either Equation 5.1 or

$$\frac{dC}{dt} = -\left(\frac{CL \cdot \left(1 + m_{CL} \cdot \sin\left(\frac{2 \cdot \pi \, t}{tp}\right)\right)}{V}\right) \cdot C + \frac{Ro}{V} \tag{5.3}$$

where m_{CL} is the fraction of clearance modulation ($0 \leq m_{CL} \leq 1$).

In Figure 5.3, when both the clearance and infusion rate are modulated, the central compartment concentration is determined by

$$\frac{dC}{dt} = -\left(\frac{CL \cdot \left(1 + m_{CL} \cdot \sin\left(\frac{2 \cdot \pi \, t}{tp} + P_{CL}\right)\right)}{V}\right) \cdot C + \frac{Ro\left(1 + \sin\left(\frac{2 \cdot \pi \, t}{tp}\right)\right)}{V} \tag{5.4}$$

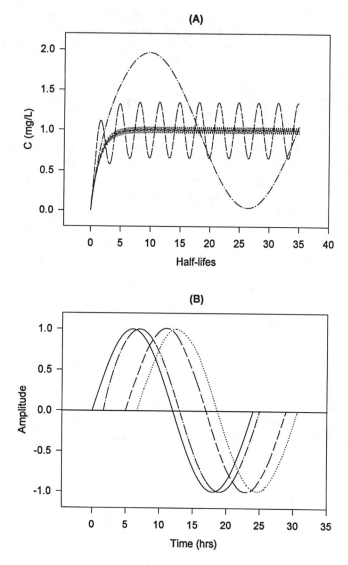

FIGURE 5.2 (A) Illustration of the influence of the time response of the central compartment on the plasma concentration achieved when the infusion rate is sinusoidally varied with a period of 24 h (tp) or held constant. The constant infusion rate equals 1 mg/h and the sinusoidally varying infusion rate is 100% modulated having an average value of 1 mg/h. In A, time is plotted in terms of the drug half-life ($t_{1/2}$). In B, plots for one period of oscillation, at steady state, are given as a function of time. In B, the phase shifts, which occur for the various $t_{1/2}$/tp ratios, are more easily visualized by only showing one infusion cycle at steady state. In A and B, the plots designated by a solid line are for a constant infusion, plots which are represented by dash–dot lines are for $t_{1/2}$/tp = 0.03, plots which are represented by dashed lines are for $t_{1/2}$/tp = 0.3, and plots which are depicted by dash-dot lines are for $t_{1/2}$/tp = 3.

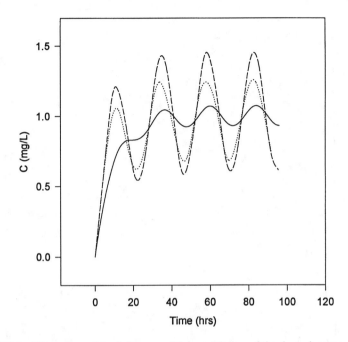

FIGURE 5.3 Illustration of the influence of the modulation of the drug clearance (CL) and the simultaneous modulation of the drug infusion rate and its clearance on the plasma concentration (C) time profile in the central compartment. In all simulations, CL = 1 L/h, V = 10 L and the infusion rate is 100% modulated having an average rate of 1 mg/h and a period of 24 h. The average value for CL and the V were chosen to represent a drug having an intermediate half-life and, thus, intermediate response time. A 20% modulation of CL is chosen, having a period of oscillation of 24 h, because these values are consistent with the experimental data.[1,5] The solid line depicts the central plasma compartment concentration as its clearance is modulated by 20%. The dashed line shows the maximum possible modulated central compartment plasma concentration obtained when both the clearance and rate of infusion are modulated. The dotted line depicts the minimum possible modulated central compartment plasma concentration obtained when both the clearance and rate of infusion are modulated. The maximum and minimum relative phase shifts were obtained through a program written in MATLAB which performs an optimal search.

where p_{CL} is the clearance phase shift ($0 \le p_{CL} \le 2\pi$ radians, i.e., $0° \le p_{CL} \le 360°$) relative to the infusion rate.

Maximum and minimum modulated plasma concentrations are obtained in Figure 5.3 by systematically varying p_{CL} and searching for the maximum and minimum modulated plasma concentrations that can be obtained. The search was accomplished by running an optimal search program developed using MATLAB.

In Figure 5.4, the central compartment plasma concentration, the effect compartment concentration and the effect are given for a constant rate of infusion and for a modulated rate of infusion. The differential equations governing this system are Equations 5.1, 5.2, and

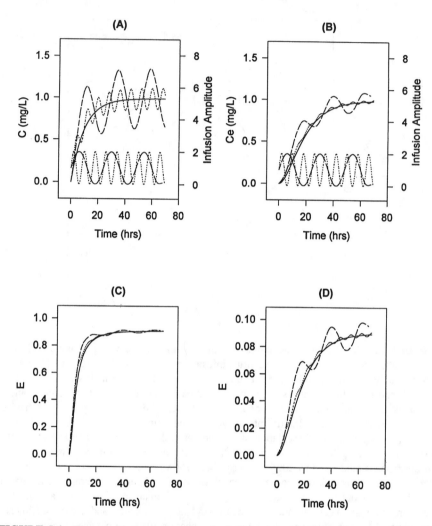

FIGURE 5.4 The graphical results, when the infusion rate is held constant or modulated 100% with a period of 24 h or for a period of 8 h, for the central plasma compartment concentration, C (A), the effect compartment concentration, Cd (B), the effect, E, when EC_{50} = 0.01 mg/L (C) and when EC_{50} = 10 mg/L (D). In all simulations, CL = 1 L/h, V = 10 L, Ve = 0.1 L, ko = 0.001 h^{-1}, ke = 0.1 h^{-1}, and γ = 1. The values for CL and the V are chosen to represent a drug having an intermediate half-life and, thus, intermediate response time. Ve is arbitrarily chosen to be 100 times smaller than V simply to reflect the fact that the effect compartments are often much smaller than V. The response time of the effect compartment is also chosen to be intermediate by setting ke equal to 0.1 h^{-1} and ko is set equal to 0.001 h^{-1} so that the mass transfer into the effect compartment would be negligible. γ is chosen to equal unity because Equation 5.6 is then consistent with a single drug molecule interacting reversibly with a receptor to produce a drug–receptor complex which then subsequently produces an effect (all microrate constants associated with this process are assumed to be first order). In C, EC_{50} is chosen to be much less than the average Ce at steady state to demonstrate the result of a saturable effect. In D, EC_{50} is chosen to be much greater than the

$$\frac{dCe}{dt} = \left(\frac{ko \cdot V}{Ve}\right) \cdot C - keo \cdot Ce \tag{5.5}$$

The effect is calculated from Ce by using Equation 5.6

$$E = \frac{E_{max} \cdot Ce^{\gamma}}{EC_{50}^{\gamma} + Ce^{\gamma}} \tag{5.6}$$

where E is the effect, E_{max} is the maximum effect, EC_{50} is the concentration at the effect site which produces 50% of the maximum effect, and γ is the shape factor.[10]

Figure 5.5 gives the results for central plasma concentration, the effect concentration, and the effect when just the clearance is modulated or the clearance and infusion rate are both simultaneously modulated. The equations governing this system are Equations 5.3 through 5.6.

Figure 5.6 shows the influence of the simultaneous modulation of the clearance and the effect response; and also for the simultaneous modulation of the clearance, infusion rate, and the effect response on the observed effect. The equations describing the system are Equations 5.3 through 5.7. Equation 5.7 describes the additional influence of a modulated receptor response, such that

$$E_m = E \cdot \left(1 + m_e \cdot \sin\left(\frac{2 \cdot \pi \cdot t}{tp} + p_e\right)\right) \tag{5.7}$$

where E_m is the receptor modulated effect, m_e is the fraction of clearance modulation ($0 \le m_e \le 1$), and p_e is the receptor response phase shift ($0 \le p_e \le 2\pi$ radians) relative to the infusion rate.

Figure 5.7 compares the central compartment plasma concentration, the effect compartment concentration, and the effect profiles obtained by modulating the infusion rate sinusoidally versus pulsing the infusion rate. The pulsed infusion rate waveform was obtained from a Fourier series expansion of the actual pulsed infusion rate profile. The Fourier series expansion of a pulsed infusion rate profile ($f(t)$)

FIGURE 5.4 (continued) average Ce at steady state to allow for maximum modulation of effect. In A and B, the upper set of three curves are plots of C as a function of t and Ce as a function of t, respectively. The solid lines represent a constant rate of infusion equal to 1 mg/h, the dashed lines are for a 100% modulated infusion rate (period equal to 24 h) having a mean value of 1 mg/h, and the dotted lines are for a 100% modulated infusion rate (period equal to 8 h) having a mean value of 1 mg/h. The lower set of two curves in A and B are the modulated infusion rate profiles, dashed line (period of 24 h) and dotted line (period of 8 h). In C and D, the solid lines represent a constant rate of infusion equal to 1 mg/h, the dashed lines are for a 100% modulated infusion rate (period equal to 24 h) having a mean value of 1 mg/h and the dotted lines are for a 100% modulated infusion rate (period equal to 8 h) having a mean value of 1 mg/h.

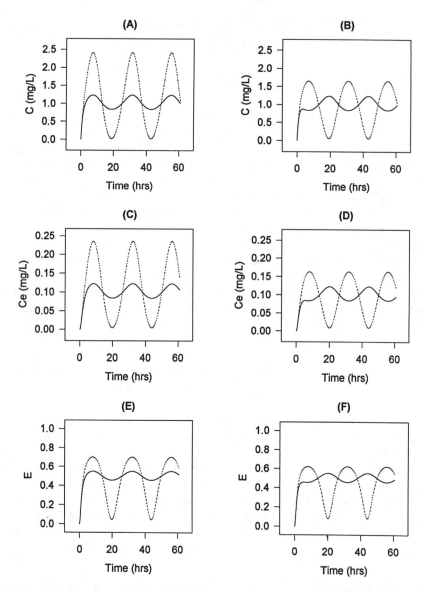

FIGURE 5.5 The influence of the modulation of the clearance (solid lines) and the simultaneous modulation of the clearance and infusion rate (dotted lines) on the concentration in the central plasma compartment (*C*), the concentration in the effect compartment (*Ce*), and on the effect (*E*). The clearance is modulated by 20% and the rate of infusion is modulated by 100%. Both the clearance and rate of infusion have an oscillation period of 24 h. A 20% modulation of CL is chosen, having a period of oscillation of 24 h, because these values are consistent with experimental data.[1,5] In all simulations, the average CL = 10 L/h, *V* = 10 L, Ve = 0.1 L, ko = 0.001 h^{-1}, ke = 1 h^{-1}, EC_{50} = 0.1 mg/L, γ = 1, and the average rate of infusion equals 1 mg/h. The average value for CL and the value for *V* are chosen to represent a drug having a short half-life and, thus, rapid response time. Ve is arbitrarily chosen to be 100 times

having minimum value of zero, an amplitude of unity, a duty cycle of $2c$, and a period of $2L$ is given by[6]

$$f(t) = \frac{c}{L} + \frac{2}{\pi}\sum_{n=1}^{\infty}\frac{(-1)^n}{n}\cdot\left(\sin\left(\frac{n\cdot\pi\cdot c}{L}\right)\right)\cdot\left(\cos\left(\frac{n\cdot\pi\cdot t}{L}\right)\right) \qquad (5.8)$$

The equations used in obtaining the data plotted in Figure 5.7 are Equations 5.1, 5.2, 5.5, 5.6, and 5.8. To obtain the results for the pulsed delivery system, $f(t)$ was substituted for $1 + \sin(2\cdot\pi\cdot t/tp)$ in Equation 5.2.

These differential equations are solved by using a series of programs written using MATLAB. The method of solution is based on an automatic step-size Runge–Kutta–Fehlberg integration method.[7]

5.4   DISCUSSION OF THE RESULTS OBTAINED FROM SIMULATIONS BASED ON THE MODEL

Figure 5.2 shows the influence of the modulation frequency on the plasma concentration time profile. Note that the amplitude of the sinusoidal portion of the concentration profile decreases as the ratio of the half-life of the drug to that of the period of the rate of infusion oscillation increases (Figure 5.2A). This is because as the half-life of the drug increases, relative to the infusion rate period, the body cannot respond to the relatively more rapid variations in the infusion rate. If, however, the half-life of the drug is decreased, either by decreasing the volume of distribution of the drug or by increasing the clearance if the drug, then the body can respond more rapidly to the changes in infusion rate and the amplitude of the sinusoidal portion of the concentration time profile will increase. Also, as the ratio of the half-life of the drug to that of the period of the rate of infusion oscillation increases, the body's response lags further behind that of the infusion (Figure 5.2B). That is, a phase shift has occurred. Therefore, to obtain a maximal modulation of the effect, the infusion must be started at a time that allows for the maximum plasma concentration to be

---

FIGURE 5.5 (continued)   smaller than V simply to reflect the fact that the effect compartments are often much smaller than V. The response time of the effect compartment is also chosen to be rapid by setting ke equal to 1 h[-1] and ko was set equal so that the mass transfer into the effect compartment would be negligible. EC_{50} is chosen to equal approximately the average Ce at steady state so that the modulation of the effect would be centered around $0.5\ E_{max}$. γ is chosen to equal unity because Equation 5.6 is then consistent with a single drug molecule interacting reversibly with a receptor to produce a drug–receptor complex which then subsequently produces an effect (all microrate constants associated with this process are assumed to be first order). In A, C, and E, the relative phase shift between the clearance and the rate of infusion has been optimized to produce the maximum effect. In B, D, and F, the relative phase shift between the clearance and the infusion rate has been optimized to produce the minimum effect. The maximum and minimum relative phase shifts are obtained through a program written in MATLAB which performs an optimal search.

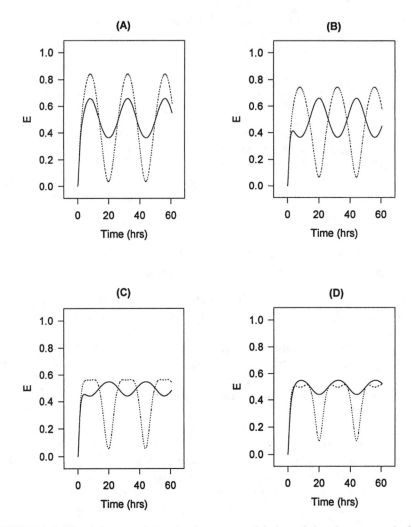

FIGURE 5.6 The influence of the simultaneous modulation of the clearance and effect response (solid lines) and also for the simultaneous modulation of the clearance, rate of infusion, and effect response (dotted lines) on the effect (E). The same pharmacokinetic parameters used to create Figure 5.5 are used. In addition, the effect response is now modulated by 20% and has an oscillation period of 24 h. A 20% modulation of effect response is chosen, having a period of oscillation of 24 h, because these values are consistent with experimental data.[1,5] A and B take the maximum possible modulated effect concentrations (shown in C) and then modulate these concentrations by a modulated effect response to produce optimally a maximum response (A) and a minimum response (B). C and D take the minimum possible modulated effect concentrations (shown in D) and then modulate these concentrations by a modulated effect response to produce optimally a maximum response (C) and a minimum response (D). The relative phase shifts required to produce the maximum and minimum responses were obtained through a program written in MATLAB which performs an optimal search.

obtained when it can ultimately result in the greatest modulation of drug efffect. Finally, note that analytical equations, based on linear systems analysis, have been derived which allow for the calculation of the concentration amplitude attenuation and phase shift responses occurring in one-to-n sequentially connected pharmaco-kinetic compartmental models as a result of a sinusoidally modulated infusion rate.[8] In addition, another interesting application of linear systems analysis to a one-compartment model having a sinusoidal infusion rate has also been published.[9]

Since the renal elimination of some drugs can undergo circadian rhythms[1,5] and certain enzymes involved in drug metabolism may also undergo circadian rhythms,[1,5] the drug clearance can sometimes undergo a circadian rhythm. Figure 5.3 illustrates that, depending on the relative phase relationship between the drug clearance and that of the infusion rate, one can obtain either constructive or destructive interference between the modulation of the rate of infusion and that of the drug clearance. This results in either a greater (constructive interference) or lower (destructive interference) in the degree of concentration modulation.

In terms of the ultimate effectiveness of a drug, it is the concentration of the drug at the effect site and the response it elicits that is of central importance. Using the model given in Figure 5.1, one can investigate the influence of modulation of the infusion rate of the drug on the concentration of drug in the effect compartment and the resulting effect produced. Figure 5.4 shows the results of a constant and a modulated infusion rate (period of 24 and 8 h) on the central compartment plasma concentration (Figure 5.4A), the effect compartment concentration (Figure 5.4B), and on the effect produced (Figure 5.4C and D). It can be observed that the lag time between the concentration effect of the compartment and the infusion is greater than that observed between the central compartment concentration and the infusion. The reason for this greater lag time is that now not only does the response time of the central compartment increase lag time, but so does the response time of the effect compartment. For the same reason, the amplitude of the sinusoidally varying component of the effect compartment decreases to a greater extent than that of the central compartment concentration. Notice that the attenuation on the amplitude and phase shift of the modulated concentration in the central compartment and the effect compartment is more pronounced when the period of the infusion rate is 8 h rather than 24 h. This is consistent with the results given in Figure 5.2. In the limiting case, as the response time of the central compartment and the effect compartment become infinitely fast, there would be no observed lag time and the amplitude of the sinusoidal variation in effect compartment concentration would be maximal. This condition would be approached when the removal of drug from both the central and effect compartments is as large as possible. Note that if the concentration in the effect compartment saturates the effect compartment response (Figure 5.4D), then modulation of the drug concentration will have little impact of the response. This can be seen by examining Equation 5.6. From Equation 5.6, we can see that if Ce is much greater than EC_{50}, then E approaches E_{max} and E is relatively independent of the value of Ce. Conversely, maximal modulation of the effect is produced when Ce is much less than EC_{50} (Figure 5.4D).

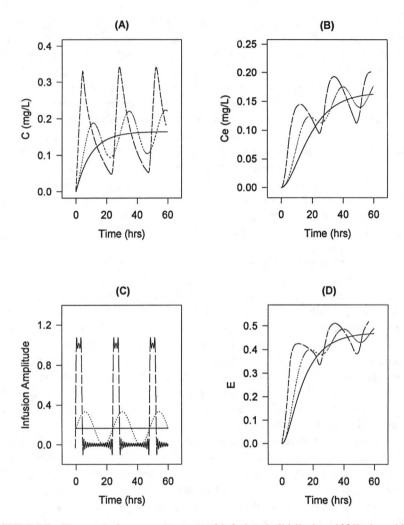

FIGURE 5.7 The result for a constant rate of infusion (solid line), a 100% sinusoidally modulated rate of infusion having a period of 24 h (dotted line) and for a pulsed rate of infusion having a duty cycle of 4 h and a period of 24 h (dashed line) on the plasma concentration of the central compartment (C), the effect concentration (Ce), and the effect (E). All rates of infusion were normalized to deliver the same amount of drug over a 24-h period. The infusion rate profiles are shown in C. The pulse waveform shown in C was constructed by taking the first 20 terms in the Fourier series expansion of the actual pulsed waveform. In all simulations CL = 1 L/h, V = 10 L, Ve = 0.1 L, ko = 0.001 h^{-1}, ke = 0.1 h^{-1}, EC_{50} = 0.185 mg/L, and γ = 1. The values for CL and the V are chosen to represent a drug having an intermediate half-life and, thus, intermediate response time. Ve is arbitrarily chosen to be 100 times smaller than V simply to reflect the fact that the effect compartments are often much smaller than V. The response time of the effect compartment is also chosen to be intermediate by setting ke equal to 0.1 h^{-1} and ko is set equal to 0.001 h^{-1} so that the mass transfer into the effect compartment would be negligible. EC_{50} was set equal to the average

The plots in Figure 5.5 demonstrate the influence of the simultaneous modulation of the drug clearance and infusion rate. Note that as in Figure 5.4 the response can either be maximized (Figure 5.5A, C, and E) or minimized (Figure 5.5B, D, and F) by adjusting the relative phase shift between the drug clearance and infusion rate. It can be observed that if constructive interference is occurring between the modulated infusion rate and clearance, then the modulation of the central plasma compartment concentration (Figure 5.5A), the effect concentration (Figure 5.5C) and the effect produced by the drug (Figure 5.5E) will be increased. Conversely, if destructive interference occurs between the modulated infusion rate and clearance then the modulation of the central compartment plasma concentration (Figure 5.5B), the effect compartment concentration (Ce) and the effect produced by the drug (Figure 5.5F) will be decreased. Once again, if the modulated effect concentration is large enough to saturate the, then little, if any, modulation of the response of the effect site will be observed.

Not only can the drug infusion rate and clearance be modulated, but the effect compartment response can also undergo a circadian rhythm.[1,5] One of the best-known examples is the fluctuation in nocturnal asthma.[5] The plots in Figure 5.6 illustrate how the observed effect is modulated by sinusoidally varying the drug clearance, infusion rate, and the receptor response with a period of 24 h. Again, if constructive interference occurs (Figure 5.6A and C), modulation of the response will be maximized, whereas if destructive interference occurs (Figure 5.6B and D), modulation of response will be minimized.

The results obtained by the sinusoidal modulation of the infusion rate can be extended to pulsed drug delivery are shown in Figure 5.7. The results of the Fourier series expansion of the pulsed infusion rate profile and for a pure sinusoidal infusion rate profile are given in Figure 5.7C. Notice that the percent modulation in the central compartment plasma concentration (Figure 5.7A), effect concentration (Figure 5.7B) and effect (Figure 5.7D) is greater for the pulsed delivery when compared with the sinusoidal delivery of drug. This trend increases as the duty cycle decreases, reaching a maximum value when the drug is periodically administered as a delta function (a bolus dose). Finally, recognize that the Fourier series expansion technique is applicable to any arbitrarily shaped periodic temporal infusion rate profile.

Total protein concentrations in the body can also undergo a circadian rhythm.[1,5] As such, one would hypothesize that if the total protein concentration is modulated, then so might the fraction of unbound drug in the body (Figure 5.8A). Strictly speaking, this is correct but whether or not it is clinically relevant depends, in part, on whether or not the drug is highly bound. If not, then modulation of protein concentration will have a decreased clinical impact. The reason for this can be seen by examination of Equation 5.9

FIGURE 5.7 (continued) Ce at steady state so that the modulation of the effect would be centered around 0.5 E_{max}. γ is chosen to equal unity because Equation 5.6 is then consistent with a single drug molecule interacting reversibly with a receptor to produce a drug–receptor complex which then subsequently produces an effect (all microrate constants associated with this process are assumed to be first order).

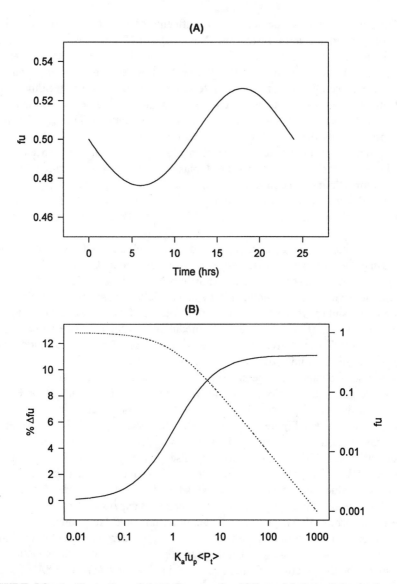

FIGURE 5.8 A, illustration of the influence of a 10% modulation of the total protein concentration on the fraction of unbound drug in the plasma (fu) having a mean value of 0.5. A 10% modulation of total plasma concentration, having a period oscillation of 24 h, was chosen because these values are consistent with experimental data.[1,5] B, a plot of the percent change in fu (%Δfu) as a function of $K_a \cdot fu_p \langle P_t \rangle$ (solid line). B also gives a plot of fu vs. $K_a \cdot fu_p \langle P_t \rangle$ (dotted line). where K_a is the association constant between the drug and plasma protein (a one-to-one association is assumed between the drug and the protein), fu_p is the fraction of total protein binding sites occupied and $\langle P_t \rangle$ is the average total concentration of plasma protein. The data used for fu were generated by using the fact that fu $= 1/(1 + K_a \cdot fu_p \langle P_t \rangle)$ (Equation 5.9).

$$fu = \frac{1}{1 + K_a fu_p P_t} \tag{5.9}$$

where K_a is the association constant (assuming only a single one to one association between the protein and drug), fu_p is the fraction of total binding sites unoccupied, and P_t is the total protein concentration.[10] Let $\langle P_t \rangle$ be the average total protein concentration. Now if $K_a fu_p \langle P_t \rangle$ is much less than 1, then modulating P_t has no effect. This would correspond to the clinical case where the drug is mostly unbound. Conversely, if $K_a fu_p \langle P_t \rangle$ is approximately equal to 1 or greater than 1, then modulation of total protein concentration will impact on the value of fu. The maximum effect on fu is approached asymptotically as $K_a fu_p \langle P_t \rangle$ approaches infinity (Figure 5.8B). Under these circumstances both the volume of distribution and the unbound concentration of the drug will be influenced. Note that at steady state the total plasma concentration of the drug is independent of the drug volume of distribution (see Equation 5.1 with $dC/dt = 0$). Therefore, the only influence a modulation of volume of distribution will have on drug concentration, at steady state, will be due to changes in the unbound concentration of the drug. This is because the unbound drug is directly proportional to fu.[10] This modulated unbound drug concentration could then modulate the observed drug effect since the unbound drug would presumably have access to the effect site.[10] Since the percent modulation of the body's protein levels is about 10%,[1] one would expect a maximum modulation of unbound concentration levels to be approximately 11% (Figure 5.8B).

If the drug is administered at the absorption site, rather than directly into the central compartment (Figure 5.1), increased lag times may be experienced. For example, variation in stomach-emptying times may delay the drug absorption since most drugs are primarily absorbed in the intestine.[10] Given the variable nature of stomach-emptying time (e.g., its dependency on the type and quantity of food which may be simultaneously ingested with the drug), one would expect more-variable results and, therefore, greater difficulty in producing a predictable modulated drug effect. Oral temporal drug administration is also complicated by the fact that gastric emptying rates undergo circadian variation.[11] Some of the variabilities (e.g., stomach emptying time) observed in the temporal administration of oral drugs can be circumvented if the absorption site is chosen to be the skin.

5.5 INTERINDIVIDUAL VARIATION

A fundamental problem facing individuals desiring to utilize temporal drug delivery to their advantage is that most of the data currently available on circadian rhythms is population data.[12] This is problematic since there are large interindividual differences in the circadian rhythms associated with the absorption, clearance, protein binding, and receptor response of a drug. The reason for the variation of circadian rhythms can be traced to such factors as interindividual differences in genetic makeup, gender, age, and disease state. Thus, for temporal drug delivery to be made truly useful the delivery rates will have to be tailor made to the individual. One approach that shows promise, in allowing for individualization of drug delivery, is by the use of marker rhythms.[12] A marker rhythm can be defined as a circadian rhythm that can be employed as a reference system for physiological, pathological, pharmacological, and therapeutic uses. An ideal marker would be one which exhibits stability and correlates well with the particular parameter being modulated. Since for the treatment of most diseases, specificity, relevance, and continuity of assessment of the marker rhythms are required, the use of a battery of marker rhythms will probably be necessary.

5.6 SUMMARY

In summary, although temporal drug delivery holds great promise in improving drug therapy in the future, it will initially most likely only be used in a rather limited number of applications. One reason for this is because to be able to use modulated drug delivery effectively the body must be able to respond rapidly to the changes in delivery rate. For this to occur, the time frame for drug distribution to the effect site, elimination, and receptor response must be shorter than the time period of periodic drug delivery. Currently, drugs are generally not designed to have these characteristics. Even if these conditions are met, one is still faced with the fact that modulation in response so far obtained has only been approximately 50%. Often, this much improvement may not be of sufficient clinical benefit to warrant the development of the drug delivery system. One notable exception to this, is in the case where drug modulation reduces drug toxicity such as has been demonstrated in the chemotherapeutic treatment certain types of cancer.[5] Finally, even if all of the above concerns are addressed, one must deal with interindividual variability. If interindividual variation is not taken into account, the results achieved through the use of temporal drug delivery will be difficult to predict. At present, the only moderately clinically useful approach to assess a patient's own circadian rhythm profile is through the use of marker rhythms,[12] which is costly and potentially a time-consuming procedure.

REFERENCES

1. Reinberg, A. and Smolensky, M. H., Circadian changes of drug disposition, *Clin. Pharmacokinet.*, 7, 401, 1982.
2. Arendt, J., Minors, D. S., and Waterhouse, J. M., Basic concepts and implications, in *Biological Rhythms in Clinical Practice*, Arendt, J., Minors, D. S., and Waterhouse, J. M., Eds., Wright, London, 1989, chap. 1.
3. Aherne, G. W., An introduction to chronopharmacology, in *Biological Rhythms in Clinical Practice*, Arendt, J., Minors, D. S., and Waterhouse, J. M., Eds., Wright, London, 1989, chap. 2.
4. Levy, G., Chronotherapeutics pharmacokinetic constraints and opportunities, *Ann. N.Y. Acad. Sci.*, 618, 116, 1991.
5. Reinberg, A. E., Concepts in chronopharmacology, *Annu. Rev. Pharmacol. Toxicol.*, 32, 51, 1992.

6. Beyer, W. H., Ed., *CRC Standard Mathematical Tables,* 28th ed., CRC Press, Boca Raton, FL, 1987, chap. 10.

7. Forsythe, G. E., Malcolm, M. A., and Moler, C. B., *Computer Methods for Mathematical Computations*, Prentice-Hall, Englewood Cliffs, NJ, 1977.

8. Burnette, R. R., Fundamental pharmacokinetic limits on the utility of using a sinusoidal drug delivery system to enhance therapy, *J. Pharmacokinet. Biopharm.*, 20, 477, 1992.

9. Theeuwes, F. and Bayne, E., Controlled-release dosage form design, in *Controlled-Release Pharmaceuticals*, Urquhart, J., Ed., American Pharmaceutical Association, Academy of Pharmaceutical Sciences, 1981, 61–93.

10. Rowland, M. and Tozer, T. N., *Clinical Pharmacokinetics: Concepts and Applications,* 2nd ed., Lea & Febiger, Philadelphia, 1989, chap. 9.

11. Sanders, S. W. and Moore J. G., Gastrointestinal chronopharmacology: physiology, pharmacology and therapeutic implications, *Pharm. Ther.*, 54, 1, 1992.

12. Reinberg, A. E. and Ashkenazi, I. E., Interindividual differences in chronopharmacologic effects of drugs: a background for individualization of chronotherapy, *Chronobiol. Int.*, 10, 449, 1993.

6 Microelectronics

Sietse Wouters

CONTENTS

6.1 INTRODUCTION

The impact of microelectronics on our daily life is easily demonstrated by means of computers, portable telephones, television, fax machines, pacemakers, etc. Since the invention of the solid state transistor, ever smaller, cheaper, more complex, and more reliable electronic systems have been developed and the end point is not yet in sight. Dedicated and general-purpose electronics have penetrated many disciplines, like office automation, industrial manufacturing, medicine, military, avionics, space exploration, automotive industry, telecommunications, and chronometry.

In the medical and pharmaceutical field, microelectronic systems are applied in the research and development area, with examples like laboratory automation, computer-assisted surgery, pacemakers, electronic capsules, and incubation techniques to study the GI tract.[1] However, if drug delivery devices are considered that are not used for research or development purposes, but that are sold to consumers, like tablets, capsules, transdermals, and suppositories, electronic control of drug delivery is only applied in a negligibly small percentage of the market. However, two important factors make it likely that sophisticated electronically controlled drug delivery devices will become more important in the future. The first factor is the progress made in the biotechnology area, leading to numerous compounds that cannot be delivered effectively using conventional drug delivery techniques. The second factor is the rapid development in the microelectronics area with respect to price, performance, size, reliability, and power consumption of microelectronic chips. As both the demand for sophisticated drug delivery devices and the availability of microelectronic systems increase, electronic control is likely to play an increasingly important role in the drug delivery area.

This chapter starts off with an overview of the current state of the art in microelectronics. The applications of microelectronics in the drug delivery area are then reviewed on the basis of infusion systems, electronic capsules, iontophoresis devices, and special devices. The chapter closes with a conclusion on the current use of microelectronics in drug delivery systems and an outlook for the future.

6.2   STATE OF THE ART IN MICROELECTRONICS

After the first working point contact transistor in 1947 and the development of silicon technology for discrete transistors through the 1950s, it became clear in the early 1960s that it was feasible to integrate several transistors together in a single piece of silicon, leading to a so-called integrated circuit (IC). Figure 6.1 shows the approximate integration density (number of transistors on one chip) and the different IC technologies developed to date. Through the 1960s, 1970s, and 1980s, technologies for medium (MSI), large (LSI), and very large scale integration (VLSI) of electronic circuits were developed.[2] Over the last 10 years, integration density still increased, but aspects like low voltage and low power circuitry have become an important issue for battery-powered portable equipment, like cordless and cellular phones and notebook and palmtop computers. The integration of sensors together with electronics in one chip[3] became an important issue, too, with applications in the automotive industry (pressure and acceleration sensors). A technology called micromachining emerged, which enables the fabrication of microelectronics and finds applications in, e.g., analytical chemistry,[4] microfluidics,[5] neural activity recording.[6] A good overview of micromachining and its applications is given by Wise and Najafi.[7]

The following paragraphs give an extremely brief and very general overview of the most important aspects that play a role in the IC development process.

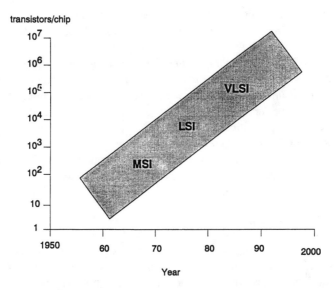

FIGURE 6.1 Graph showing the integration density of the different IC technologies as a function of time.

6.2.1 CIRCUIT DESIGN AND SIMULATION

In digital chip development, systems are composed of modular building blocks, available from a library. Examples of digital building blocks are flip-flops, registers, memory modules, arithmetic and logic units, and complete microprocessors. In analog chip development, the building block approach is also applied, but, quite often, the system constraints require that a module be adapted or that an optimized subcircuit be designed from scratch. Examples of analog building blocks are amplifiers, filters, and D/A and A/D converters. These analog and digital building blocks can usually be split up in subblocks, subsubblocks, and often in even more hierarchical levels before the transistor level is reached. A designer has to verify thoroughly that a designed circuit functions correctly before it is fabricated (due to the very high initial cost of fabrication). As a result of that, several types of simulation tools have been developed, each optimized for a different hierarchical level. Device simulation software is available (frequently based on finite element modeling) to test the behavior of a single transistor. Circuit simulation software has been developed for the simulation of small to medium-sized circuits. The main application of these simulators is in analog circuit design. High-level simulation software is available for the simulation of large and complex circuits; the main application is for digital circuitry. These simulators use very simple transistor models, so that the simulation speed is very high, which makes it possible to simulate large circuits in a reasonable time. Besides simulation tools, design software is available to generate layouts of single transistors up to complete microprocessors. The approach used most frequently is the one in which a library with modules is available. Designers can take the models from the library and use them in their design. Placing a number of modules in an optimal configuration and making the connections between them can be a time-consuming and tedious task, which is usually taken over by automatic route-and-place software. After the route-and-place procedure, the parasitic elements (e.g., when two metal lines cross one another, a parasitic capacitance is created) can be calculated. Once a complete circuit has been composed and the layout generated, its digital and/or analog functionality and its frequency response are simulated. Besides checking the functionality of the system, as well as temperature dependence, the influence of its parasitic elements and the effects of variations in the process parameters are evaluated. When the simulation outcome is not in accordance with the desired circuit performance, the design and simulation process is repeated in an iterative way until the desired circuit performance is achieved. Only then is the design ready for chip fabrication.

6.2.2 CHIP FABRICATION

The fabrication of silicon chips takes place in a series of usually 20 to 30 processing steps in a cleanroom environment. For each processing step, a photolithographic mask is required, usually with a submicrometer resolution. The processing steps for IC's include, e.g., thermal oxidation and diffusion, ion implantation, wet chemical etching, plasma etching, polysilicon and aluminum deposition. Since the cleanroom environment and the photolithography and processing equipment are all very capital intensive, chip fabrication is associated with an extremely high nonrecurrent engineering (NRE) cost. On the other hand, the materials cost per chip is extremely low (usually <50 mm^2 monocrystalline silicon). This means that microelectronic chip production is only profitable when huge numbers are produced and the NRE cost is shared by millions or billions of devices. During the 1960s, 1970s, and 1980s only large electronics companies could make the large investments necessary for chip development and production. However, in recent years, several companies and research institutes have set up programs to enable small and medium-sized companies to develop their own microelectronic devices. Basically, the design tools are offered on a lease basis or PC-based tools are available, whereas the development cost is kept low by sharing the NRE cost among several users. This approach is called "multi project wafer service": several layouts from different customers are processed together, so that the mask costs and the fabrication costs are shared among the customers. This means that at this moment, even small and medium-sized companies can afford to develop their own application-specific IC and have it produced in relatively small numbers.

6.2.3 DEVICE PACKAGING

Conventionally, DIL (duel in-line) packages are used for encapsulation of chips. The chip is placed on a substrate and bonded using thin gold or aluminum wires ($\varnothing$ 25 μm), as shown in Figure 6.2. Either a ceramic package with a hermetically sealed cover (high quality, high price) or an injection molded package (lower quality, low price) is used. These DIL packages are used in so-called through-hole technology, in which the pins of the devices are put through the board, as shown in the left

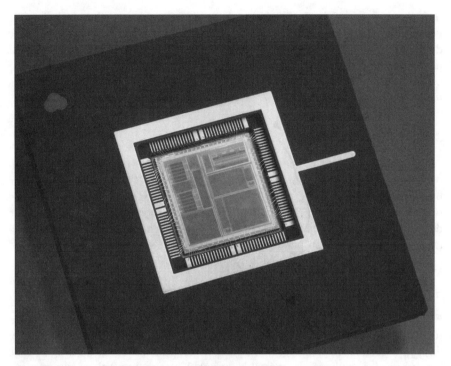

FIGURE 6.2   Photograph of a 14-pin ceramic DIL package without cover. It clearly shows the silicon chip (3×3 mm^2) and the aluminum bond wires (25 μm diameter).

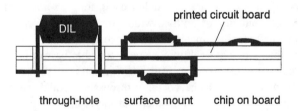

FIGURE 6.3   Schematic drawing showing the different techniques to package ICs and to mount them on a printed circuit board.

part of Figure 6.3. In through-hole technology, one side of the board contains (most of) the components, whereas (most of) the interconnection pattern is on the other side. The continuing demand for smaller packages and higher pin counts led to the development of surface-mount devices, which use two (like DIL) or four rows of pins or which have a pin grid array under the complete package. In surface-mount technology, components can be placed on both sides of the board. Boards are usually made of many insulating layers, between which additional interconnect layers can be defined. A schematic drawing of a multilayered printed circuit board using surface-mount technology is shown in the middle part of Figure 6.3. One step further in packaging technology is the chip-on-board (COB) technique, in which the chip is placed directly on the circuit board or in the system. The bare chip is wire-bonded directly to the board, as shown in the right part of Figure 6.3. This technology is used for a variety of applications, one of the most interesting examples being chip cards, in which the chip, including readout contacts, is packaged in a 0.8-mm-thick plastic card.

6.3 INFUSION SYSTEMS

Commercially available infusion systems can be classified as ambulatory or nonambulatory, extracorporeal or implantable, and as systems of which the pump is driven by mechanical, chemical, electrical, elastomeric, or other types of energy. A good overview is given by Tyle.[8] Typical application for infusion systems are, e.g., insulin delivery, chemotherapy, and analgesia. Since this chapter focuses on the microelectronic aspects of infusion pumps, we will concentrate on electronically controlled ambulatory and implantable infusion systems.

6.3.1 EXTRACORPOREAL AMBULATORY INFUSION SYSTEMS

Extracorporeal ambulatory infusion systems usually have the size of a cigarette box (or somewhat larger, depending on the drug volume), and they have a catheter through which the drug is infused. The pump mechanism that drives the drug through the catheter is usually of the peristaltic, solenoid, electrochemical, or syringe type. All of the electronically controlled infusion systems contain a microprocessor, a ROM module containing the system software and a RAM module for storing the user-defined parameters. The electronic units are usually constructed using standard off-the-shelf components and are assembled using through-hole or surface-mount technology or a combination of both. A wide variety of extracorporeal ambulatory systems are available[9] from companies like Cormed, Pharmacia, Pancretec, and Medfusion. Most of the extracorporeal pumps are intended to be worn in a pocket or on a belt. One exception is the Panoject from Elan, which is an infusion system with a wrist strap that is worn like a watch. A detailed discussion of all these infusion systems would be beyond the scope of this chapter and therefore only one example is discussed, one that deviates significantly from the average ambulatory infusion system.

6.3.1.1 DeBio Tech, Chronojet

The Chronojet is an ambulatory infusion system developed by DeBio Tech, Lausanne, Switzerland. This system has two unique features. First, this ambulatory infusion system is the first device using a pump manufactured by micromachining techniques.[5] The pump itself is shown in Figure 6.4, it measures $20 \times 10 \times 3$ mm^3 and administers volumes ranging from 0.1 µL to 150 mL per day. The second special feature is that the whole Chronojet is designed to be disposed of after about 8 days of operation. This is made possible through the use of silicon fabrication technology for the electronics and the pump, so that the total price can be kept relatively low when large volumes are produced.

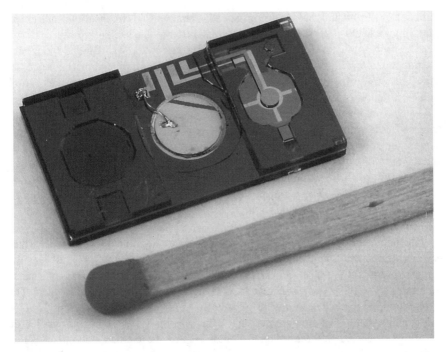

FIGURE 6.4   Photograph of a silicon micropump used in the infusion system by DeBio Tech.

6.3.2   IMPLANTABLE INFUSION SYSTEMS

Only a few implantable infusion systems have been developed that are commercially available today. Usually, these devices are implanted in the abdominal region, whereas the drug-delivering catheter tip is led to the spot where the drug dosing is required. Two types of pumping mechanisms are applied in implantable pumps: peristaltic and solenoid. Since the size and weight of the pump play a more important role than the price (the implantation is usually the most expensive part), dedicated ICs are usually applied in implantable infusion systems.

Major problems associated with implantable infusion pumps are biocompatibility, reliability, and operational lifetime of battery and electronics; the use of concentrated drugs; clogging of the catheter, etc. In order to get a good idea of the microelectronic systems used to control implantable pumps, one infusion system is discussed here in detail.

6.3.2.1   Medtronic, SynchroMed Programmable Pump

The Medtronic Drug Administration System (DAS) consists of an implantable drug administration device (DAD) with a catheter and an extracorporeal telemetric programming unit. A general description of this system is given in Chapter 9 of this book. In this section, we will focus on the microelectronic system of the DAD. The complete electronic unit basically consists of an antenna and two custom-made chips, one digital CMOS processor chip, and one analog bipolar telemetry chip.

The processor chip has an 8-bit architecture, runs at approximately 33 kHz, and is equipped with 112 bytes RAM and 2 kbytes ROM, all integrated on the processor chip. This custom-made processor chip was purposely designed with a rather simple architecture, low clock frequency, and limited memory capacity in order to minimize power consumption and thus maximize operational lifetime. On the other hand, the processor is powerful enough to control a variety of drug delivery profiles consisting of up to ten consecutive time segments, to store information on the pump, the patient, and the currently used drug, and to check continuously for several alarm conditions. The most important function of the processor is to execute the drug-dosing program and control the peristaltic pump. The last is achieved by sending digital pulses directly from the processor chip to the stepper motor of the peristaltic pump, which proceeds one step upon every pulse.

The telemetry chip contains a transmitter–receiver circuit and forms the interface between the antenna and the processor chip. The DAD antenna is a coil and the external programming head contains a similar coil. Communication can take place by bringing the two coils close together, so that they are inductively coupled. The information is transmitted by means of radiofrequency magnetic fields. The DAD is hermetically sealed in a titanium housing, which shields the electronics from electric fields, but is transparent for the magnetic fields used for the telemetric communication. In order to prevent accidentally occurring magnetic fields from disturbing the running program, a reed switch must be activated to connect the antenna to the telemetry chip. This reed switch can be activated by a permanent magnetic field.

The two chips and a few additional components (oscillator crystal, capacitors) are mounted on a ceramic substrate using surface-mount technology. The total electronic system occupies only a small fraction of the total DAD volume and is one of the most reliable components of the DAD.

6.3.2.2   Other Implantable Infusion Systems

At Johns Hopkins University in Laurel, MD, a Programmable Implantable Medication System (PIMS) has been developed.[10] This system is commercially available from MiniMed Technologies, Sylmar, CA. Infusaid in Norwood, MA, also has developed an electronically controlled implantable infusion pump. Although the applications for the three infusion systems mentioned in this section are quite different, their sizes, construction, and electronic control units are rather similar.

6.3.3   Summary

Several types of extracorporeal and implantable infusion systems are currently available, in which the drug delivery pattern is controlled by a microprocessor. Implantable systems make full use of microelectronics technology and employ custom-made low-power integrated circuitry. In extracorporeal infusion systems, usually standard surface-mount technology is used and only a few devices use custom-made advanced microelectronic control systems.

6.4 ELECTRONIC CAPSULES

Within a decade after the invention of the solid state transistor, people came up with ideas on how to reap the benefits from these very small electronic elements. Zworykin and Farrar[11] were among the first to publish a journal article about a "radio pill" that measured pressure in the GI tract and sent out the data to an external receiver using a small, one-transistor transmitter. Almost simultaneously, Jacobson and Mackay[12,13] published their "pH endoradiosonde", which was a swallowable capsule measuring pH while traveling through the GI tract. These first devices consisted of a one-transistor oscillator, the frequency of which was modulated by the measurand. Of course, these devices did not deliver a drug, but they demonstrated that it was already possible back in 1957 to include a power source, an electronic circuit, and a sensor in a capsule that was small enough to be swallowed and to travel through the GI tract.

Between 1957 and now, many publications have appeared on electronic capsules for measuring pH,[14] temperature,[15] redox potential,[16] pressure, or GI motility,[17] for taking samples from the GI tract,[18] for performing biopsies,[19] and for drug delivery.[20] All of these electronic capsules find their applications in medical and biopharmaceutical research. The following paragraphs present some examples of the various electronic capsules that have been developed for drug delivery.

6.4.1 HF CAPSULE

In the early 1980s, Schuster and Hugemann[21] developed a remote-controlled high-frequency (HF) capsule for application in bioavailability studies. After the capsule is swallowed by a test person, it is tracked during its GI transit using X-rays. At the moment it reaches the desired location, a HF electromagnetic (EM) field is switched on, which is received by a coil antenna (1 in Figure 6.5) in the capsule. The received energy heats up a heating wire (3), which melts a nylon thread (4). This thread releases a plunger (6), which is forced by a spring (5) into a latex balloon (10). In this way, the balloon is ruptured and releases the drug with which is had been filled prior to administration. As can be observed from Figure 6.5, approximately half of the 28-mm-long and 12-mm-wide capsule volume is available for drug storage, whereas the rest is occupied by the release mechanism.

Advantages of the capsule are that there is no battery in the device. Disadvantages are that the capsule is relatively expensive, that X-rays must be applied to localize the capsule, and that a high-power HF field must be applied to release the drug. HF capsules and the telemetric equipment are commercially available from PAZ, Frankfurt am Main, Germany.

6.4.2 TELEMETRIC SHUTTLE

During the 1980s, Lambert and co-workers[19] developed the so-called autonomous telemetric capsule for application in medical and biopharmaceutical research. This capsule has a modular construction and consists of a main body and an interchangeable tip, as shown in Figure 6.6. The cylindrical main body contains two batteries

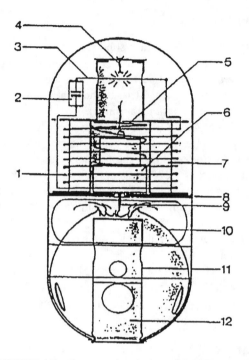

FIGURE 6.5   Cross-sectional view of the HF capsule.

and a small electronic circuit, and it provides a cavity in which a cogwheel is present. A gelatin ring covers the cavity and keeps the cogwheel inside. After the capsule has been swallowed and has reached the stomach, the gelatin ring dissolves and the cogwheel is turned and pushed out of the cavity by means of a spring and takes the position as shown in Figure 6.6. The length of the capsule is 39 mm, which prevents it from turning around in the small intestine. Hence, the capsule is propelled by the GI contents through the small intestine, while the cogwheel is pressed against the lumen wall and thus turned around during motion. One of the teeth of the cogwheel contains a small permanent magnet, which induces a signal in the magnetic sensor located near the base of the cogwheel unit. The signal from the magnetic sensor modulates the frequency of a Colpits oscillator, which frequency (around 110 MHz) is transmitted to an external receiver. The Colpits oscillator consists of one transistor and a few resistors and capacitors and is realized on an 8×12 mm^2 substrate using surface-mount components. The tuning coil of the oscillator is wound around the perimeter of the substrate and consequently functions as the antenna. Because the frequency of this relatively simple transmitter depends on its load impedance and since this load impedance depends on the distance from the capsule to the skin, which continuously changes during GI transit, the externally received frequency shows a significant drift during experiments. In order to deal with this, the external receiver has a wide-range automatic frequency control, so that it stays tuned to the capsule. The total power consumption of the electronic circuitry is 3.6 mW, which gives the transmitter a range of 15 m. Because the transmission is highly directive,

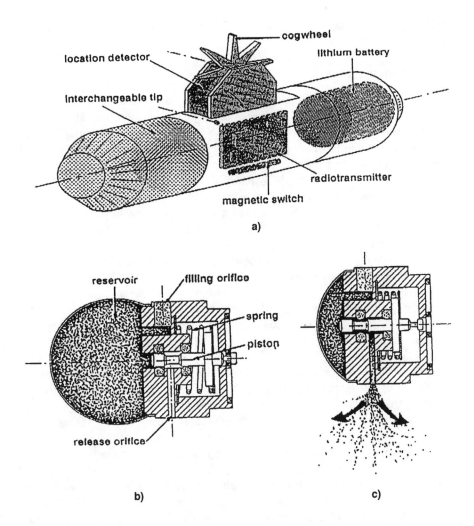

FIGURE 6.6 (a) Drawing of the telemetric shuttle, clearly showing the cogwheel, the battery, the electronic unit, and the interchangeable tip. (b) Drug release tip when filled, and (c) during release of the drug.

a range of approximately 2 m is advised for reliable communication. The accuracy of the distance measurement in the small intestine is approximately a few centimeters. The tip of the capsule is interchangeable, and different tips are available for fluid aspiration, drug delivery, and biopsies. The tip can be activated by holding a permanent magnet close to the abdomen of the patient, so that a magnetic switch is activated (just like the reed switch in the implantable DAD from Medtronic).

Advantages of this type of capsule are that it autonomously and accurately measures the distance in the small intestine and that it is very versatile because of its modular structure. Disadvantages are its large size (39 mm to prevent turning around in the small intestine) and the batteries contained in the device. Telemetric shuttles and the associated telemetric equipment is commercially available from ABS, St. Dié in France.

6.4.3 OTHER ELECTRONIC CAPSULES

In addition to the three examples discussed above, numerous electronically controlled drug delivery capsules have been developed, some of which are definitely worth mentioning. One of the most well known electronic capsules is the Heidelberg pH capsule,[22] which has been used for many biopharmaceutical studies. A unique aspect of the Heidelberg capsule is that it is powered by a battery that consists of a zinc and silver chloride electrode inserted in a reservoir that is filled with physiological saline solution prior to use. This makes the device a self-powered, but very safe device. A capsule with a release mechanism based on electrophoresis has been developed at the University of Münster in Germany. This capsule consists of an open-ended tube, filled with a drug containing hydrogel.[23,24] An electrode is inserted in the gel. A reference electrode is located at the other end of the tube. Between the two electrodes, a hermetically sealed battery compartment is located. When the battery is connected to the two electrodes, electrophoresis takes place and an ionic current flows from the first electrode, through the gel and the GI contents, to the reference electrode. In this way, the ionic drug is forced out of the gel-filled reservoir at a rate proportional to the electric current. Pulsatile release can be achieved by switching the battery on and off.

Another very interesting drug delivery capsule has been developed by the Research Triangle Institute and Glaxo.[25] It consists of two sleeves making up a drug reservoir, that can be opened and closed by means of a shape memory alloy actuator. The two sleeves have oblong holes, so that the capsule can be opened (aligning the holes) and closed by rotating one of the sleeves with respect to the other. Rotation of the sleeves is achieved by means of heating or cooling a shape memory alloy actuator by means of a telemetric link, similar to the approach used for the HF capsule. Another type of electronic drug delivery capsule has been developed by the company Gastro Target.[26] This capsule contains a battery and a small IC containing a transmitter/receiver unit. The transmitter continuously sends out EM waves, which are received by seven antennas sewn into a vest worn by the patient. By using the seven received signals, the exact position of the capsule can be calculated, and, when the capsule is at the right position, a trigger signal can be sent out. This trigger signal is received by the capsule and an electrochemical drug release mechanism is activated that drives the drug out of the capsule. Finally, Matsushita developed a capsule with a pH sensor and a small electronic circuit.[27] Upon measuring a certain pH profile, the circuit activates the release mechanism, which consists of a spring and a plunger, the last of which forces the drug out of the drug reservoir.

6.4.4 SUMMARY

Several types of electronically controlled drug delivery capsules have been developed and are commercially available for clinical studies on drug delivery or on the measurement of parameters in the GI tract. It is striking, however, that the miniaturization potential of microelectronics and micromachining has not yet been exploited to a large extent in this field. Especially, the use of integrated control electronics, micro-valves, micropumps, and the cointegration of electronics and sensors (for, e.g., pH or redox potential) could significantly improve the performance of these systems.

6.5   IONTOPHORESIS

Iontophoresis is the enhanced transport of an ionic or a nonionic compound through skin by means of an electrical voltage or current. The therapeutic relevance of this drug delivery technique is discussed in Chapters 2 and 5 of this book. The basic electrical function of an iontophoresis device is to generate a constant or time-varying current or voltage.

Usually, iontophoresis devices control the current rather than the voltage, mainly because there is a linear relation between electric current density and drug flux, so that the drug flow can be controlled by controlling the current. Current densities applied in iontophoresis usually vary between $10\ \mu A/cm^2$ and $1\ mA/cm^2$. Below this interval, the drug flux is usually too low. Above this interval, the skin is likely to be irreversibly damaged and pain is experienced by the patient. The threshold for sensation of the current is generally accepted to be around 100 to $200\ \mu A/cm^2$. Sizes of iontophoresis patches vary from a few square centimeters to approximately $100\ cm^2$. Hence, the total current roughly varies between $50\ \mu A$ and $10\ mA$. The resistance of human skin *in vivo* varies between persons and between application sites, and it decreases when iontophoresis is applied. Practically, human skin resistance values can vary from approximately $1\ k\Omega/cm^2$ to $100\ k\Omega/cm^2$. The voltage U developed across a piece of skin of resistance R upon application of current density I is given by:

$$U = RI$$

When a current density of $I = 200\ \mu A/cm^2$ is applied over a series connection of two pieces of skin (at the drug and at the reference electrode) of resistance $R = 100\ k\Omega/cm^2$, the resulting voltage is 40 V. It is important that the electronic system can accommodate these high voltage requirements.

Although much has been published on the administration of a variety of compounds using iontophoresis, only a few publications have appeared on the systems used for iontophoretic drug delivery.[28,29] Without trying to provide a complete overview of the available iontophoresis devices, two representative examples of commercially available iontophoresis systems will be discussed.

6.5.1   IOMED

The Phoresor iontophoresis system is sold by Iomed in Salt Lake City, UT. It is a tabletop, microprocessor-controlled system. In this section, we will concentrate on the electronic aspects of this device.

The heart of the Phoresor is an 8-bit microprocessor, which is equipped with 8 kbyte ROM to store the iontophoresis program and 256 bytes RAM to store the experimental data. A transformer and a rectifier circuit is used to step up the 9-V battery voltage to 80 V (DC/DC conversion) and to isolate the output leads galvanically from the rest of the system. Stepping up the battery voltage to a supply voltage of 80 V is necessary to deal with high skin impedances, as explained above. Two turning knobs are provided to adjust the desired total dose and the current level (0 to 4 mA in steps of 0.1 mA). An 8-bit D/A converter converts the digital information on the current level into a constant current. During operation, the current through the voltage across the iontophoresis electrodes are continuously monitored. As soon as a high impedance situation (e.g., loose electrode) or a low impedance situation (electrodes placed on damaged skin, skin burns as a result of too high current density) is detected, the current is automatically turned down and an alarm message is sounded and displayed. The operator must correct the alarm condition and subsequently restart the system. Since a fast change in current (dI/dt) or voltage (dV/dt) causes sensation or pain, the Phoresor has a preprogrammed limit to the temporal change in the current or voltage. If the current is increased too rapidly, audible and visible alarms are generated and the current rise is paused. After a short interval, the current can be increased further.

The current version of the Phoresor (PM 700) has been on the market since 1988 and is realized in a plastic tabletop housing with a dose- and current-level knob and an LCD display, indicating the remaining dose, the remaining time, and the current level. The circuit is realized using off-the-shelf through-hole components.

6.5.2 EMPI

The DUPEL iontophoresis system marketed by Empi in St. Paul, MN, has a structure similar to the Phoresor from Iomed. The main difference is that it is a dual-channel device. One 8-bit microprocessor controls two independent channels, each of which can be adjusted to a DC current between 0.5 and 4 mA in steps of 0.1 mA. The device measures the iontophoresis current as a feedback signal, and, when a high impedance load is detected, the current is switched off. The device does not check for a low impedance state or for fast changes in current or voltage.

The current version of the DUPEL iontophoresis system, which has been marketed since 1993, has the size of a cigarette box and is realized using off-the-shelf components, partially surface mount and partially through-hole. The same parameters can be set as in the Phoresor (total dose and current level), but the actual programming is a little more complicated because of the dual-channel configuration.

6.5.3 OTHER DEVICES

In addition to the iontophoresis devices discussed above, which are intended for delivering a drug, there are several devices on the market that send a constant or time-varying current through the skin or apply a voltage over the skin without delivering a drug. 3M markets the Dental Electronic Anesthesia System. This is an electronic device the size of a cigarette box, to which a cable with two skin electrodes (containing a gel without drug) can be connected. The device generates a square wave with an adjustable frequency in kilohertz range. The square wave is balanced around zero, which means that the signal has no DC component, so that no net current flow occurs from one of the electrodes to the other. The anesthetizing effect is attributed purely to the electrical impulses. Advance sells a self-contained system for muscle relaxation. Its working mechanism is the same as the one described above for the 3M device. Tapper[30] from Medical Device Corp. has developed several iontophoresis devices, among others an antiperspirant system.

6.5.4 SUMMARY

Commercially available iontophoresis devices are ambulatory systems that are assembled with standard electronic components using through-hole or surface-mount technology. If iontophoresis systems used custom-made ICs, they would be much smaller and more user-friendly. However, since iontophoresis is a noninvasive technique, the driving force toward system integration is much weaker for iontophoresis than it is for, e.g., implantable infusion systems.

6.6   SPECIAL DEVICES

In this section on special devices, two systems are discussed that do not deliver a drug, but that are related to drug delivery. These devices make use of and clearly demonstrate the potential of microelectronics for medical and pharmaceutical applications.

6.6.1   MEDICATION EVENT MONITORING

The company APREX in Fremont, CA, markets a medication event monitor, which consists of a regular plastic vial, used in retail pharmacy, whose closure is replaced by a special closure, which contains microelectronic circuitry.

The main application of the medication event monitor is in clinical trials. The patient receives the vial with medication and a cleared memory. During or after the therapy, the physician reads out the data stored in the memory (up to 1800 medication events) and correlates them with, e.g., the biopharmaceutical data. Another application of the medication event monitor comes in the form of a service provided by APREX. Patients with compliance problems use the medication event monitor, which is in a telemetric way connected to a modem. Over this modem connection, APREX checks patients (at home) on their compliance and warns them if the prescribed administration regimen is not carried out correctly.

The electronic circuit is realized on a circular circuit board that fits in the vial closure and that is separated from the medication. The core of the electronic system consists of a Seiko microprocessor chip and a memory chip. Both chips are directly attached to the circuit board (COB) in order to save weight and space. The chips are low-power/low-voltage devices and are working on a 3-V lithium button cell battery (18 months operational lifetime). During or after the treatment, the memory contents can be read using a noncontact communication technique. The data communication protocol is designed to be robust, in order to prevent EM interference, and it is protected against data manipulation and unintended use of the data. The basic electronic system is of general nature and could therefore easily be adapted to other pharmaceutical packages or dosage forms, like blister packages, liquid dispensers, or inhalers.

It must be noted that the vial can be opened and closed without the patient taking his or her medication, thus leading to erroneous compliance data. However, the most important aspects in patient compliance are the delay and the omission of doses, and these two events are registered correctly by the medication event monitor.

6.6.2 REGISTRATION AND MONITORING OF ANIMALS

In several countries, pets and cattle are registered with a number programmed in a transponder (8 to 40 mm length, 2 to 5 mm diameter). This transponder is injected in the animal with a large-size syringe. The transponder contains a microelectronic chip with a registration number and a coil, which picks up information and energy from an external transmitter/receiver. The transponder responds by modulating the EM waves with its information (the registration number). The modulated wave is picked up by the receiver, and, in this way, the animal is identified. Transponders are also available in a (credit) card format for goods identification in an industrial environment and for security applications to admit people to, e.g., buildings or ski lifts. More-sophisticated transponders, that are equipped with sensors, are currently being developed. An example of such a miniaturized telemetric measurement system is a pressure-sensing device that can be implanted intraocularly.[31] Other examples come from stock farming and cattle breeding, where advanced versions of the registration type of transponders are currently under development to measure parameters like temperature, blood pressure, heart rate, or activity.[32,33] These systems are not drug delivery devices as such, but complete the automated feedback loop in a health-monitoring system.

6.7 CONCLUSION

The development and production of microelectronic systems is no longer just the realm of only a few multinational companies specialized in electronics. Rather, it has become quite accessible and affordable for nonelectronics companies and for small and medium-sized industries. Microelectronic control has the potential to improve drug delivery devices, like infusion systems, electronic capsules, and iontophoresis devices, with respect to size, weight, performance, reliability, and operational lifetime. Only in implantable infusion pumps have the benefits of microelectronics been fully utilized. In electronic capsules and iontophoresis devices, microelectronic systems are not (yet) applied, but rather standard electronic components and surface-mount technology are used.

As stated in the introduction to this chapter, the rapid developments in microelectronics lead to ever smaller and more complex systems for ever lower prices, whereas the progress in biotechnology leads to effective and potent therapeutic compounds that are difficult to administer using conventional methods. These two factors, plus the fact that dedicated and general-purpose electronics have been successfully implemented in some drug delivery systems, make it very likely that microelectronics will play an increasingly important role in the drug delivery devices of the future.

ACKNOWLEDGMENT

I would like to acknowledge my colleagues, who helped me in obtaining an overview of the electrically controlled drug delivery area, and I would like to thank several people in drug delivery companies for providing data on their products.

REFERENCES

1. Antonin, K. H., Other methods in studying colonic drug absorption, in *Colonic Drug Absorption and Metabolism,* Bieck, P. R., Ed., Marcel Dekker, New York, 1993, Chap. 5.
2. Mead, C. and Conway, L., *Introduction to VLSI Systems,* Addison-Wesley, Reading, MA, 1980.
3. Middelhoek, S. and Audet, S. A., *Silicon Sensors,* Academic Press, London, 1989.
4. Manz, A., Harrison, D. J., Verpoorte, E., and Widmer, H. M., Planar chips technology for miniaturization of separation systems: a developing perspective in chemical monitoring, in *Advances in Chromatography,* 33, Brown, P. R. and Grushka, E., Eds., Marcel Dekker, New York, 1993, Chap. 1.
5. van de Pol, F. C. M., van Lintel, H. T. G., Elwenspoek, M., and Fluitman, J. H. J., A thermopneumatic micropump based on micro-engineering techniques, *Sensors Actuators,* A21-23, 198, 1990.
6. Hoogerwerf, A. C. and Wise, K. D., A three dimensional neural recording array, *Digest IEEE International Conference on Solid State Sensors and Actuators,* 120, 1991.
7. Wise, K. D. and Najafi, K., Microfabrication techniques for integrated sensors and microsystems, *Science,* 254, 1335, 1991.
8. Tyle, P., Ed., *Drug Delivery Devices,* Marcel Dekker, New York, 1988.
9. Lukacsko, P. and May, G. S., Ambulatory infusion devices, in *Drug Delivery Devices,* Tyle, P., Ed., Marcel Dekker, New York, 1988, Chap. 5.
10. Fischell, R. E., A programmable implantable medication system (PIMS) as a means for intracorporeal drug delivery, in *Drug Delivery Devices,* Tyle, P., Ed., Marcel Dekker, New York, 1988, Chap. 8.
11. Zworykin, V. K. and Farrar, J. T., A "radio pill," *Nature,* 179, 898, 1957.
12. Mackay, R. S. and Jacobson, B., Endoradiosonde, *Nature,* 179, 1239, 1957.
13. Jacobson, B. and Mackay, R. S., A pH-endoradiosonde, *Lancet,* 1, 1224, 1957.
14. Evans, D. F., Pye, G., Bramley, R., Clark, A. G., Dyson, T. J., and Hardcastle, J. D., Measurement of gastrointestinal pH profiles in normal ambulent human subjects, *Gut,* 29(8), 1035, 1988.
15. Cutchis, P. N., Hogrefe, A. F., and Lesho, J. C., The ingestible thermal monitoring system, *Johns Hopkins APL Tech. Dig.,* 9(1), 16, 1988.
16. Stirrup, V., Ledingham, S. J., Thomas, M., Pye, G., and Evans, D. F., Redox potential measurement in the gastrointestinal tract in man, *Gut,* 31, A1171, 1990.
17. Thorburn, H. A., Carter, K. B., Goldberg, J. A., and Finlay, I. G., Remote control systems' radiotelemetry receiver 7060: its use in clinical colonic motility measurement, *J. Med. Eng. Technol.,* 13(5), 252, 1989.
18. Pochart, P., Lémann, F., Flourié, B., Pellier, P., Goderel, I., and Rambaud, J. C., Pyxigraphic sampling to enumerate methanogens and anaerobes in the right colon of healthy humans, *Gastroenterology,* 105, 1281, 1993.
19. Lambert, A., Vaxman, F., Crenner, F., Wittmann, T., and Grenier, J. F., Autonomous telemetric capsule to explore the small bowel, *Med. Biol. Eng. Computing,* 191, 1991.

20. Staib, A. H., Woodcock, B. G., Loew, D., and Schuster, O., Remote control of gastrointestinal drug delivery in man, in *Novel Drug Delivery and Its Therapeutic Application,* Prescott, L. F. and Nimmo, W. S., Eds., John Wiley, Chichester, U.K., 1989, Chap. 8, pp. 79–88.

21. Schuster, O. and Hugemann, B., Course of development of the HF-capsule — variations and method-related typical findings, in *Proc. International Workshop on Methods in Clinical Pharmacology,* Rietbrock, N., Woodcock, B. G., Staib, H., and Loew, D., Eds., Frankfurt, 28, 1986.

22. Heidelberg Capsule, *World Medical Electronics,* 150, 1964.

23. Gröning, R., Schrader, D., and Schwarze, S., Microelectronic control circuits to control the release of drugs from dosage forms, *Pharm. Pharmacol. Lett.,* 1, 29, 1991.

24. Gröning, R., Schrader, D., and Schwarze, S., Pulsatile release of flupenthixol from dosage forms by electrical fields, *Pharm. Pharmacol. Lett.,* 1, 49, 1991.

25. Glanz, J., Robot pill helps the medicine go down, *R&D Biosci. Pharm.,* 35(6), 73, 1993.

26. D'Andrea, D. T., Adelman, M. H., and Shentag, J. J., A new method for site-specific delivery in the gastrointestinal (GI) tract, *Proc. AAPS Meeting,* CS 3017, 1991.

27. Matsushita, Japanese Patent Application 5 8194 809, 1982.

28. Zakzewski, C. A. and Li, J. K. L., Design of a novel constant current pulsed iontophoretic stimulation device, in *Proc. 18th IEEE Annual Northeast Bioengineering Conference,* Ohley, W. J., Ed., Kingston, RI, 33, 1992.

29. Jaw, F.-S., Wang, C.-Y., and Huang, Y.-Y., Portable current stimulator for transdermal iontophoretic drug delivery, *Med. Eng. Phys.,* 17(5), 385, 1995.

30. Tapper, R., Design of an electronic antiperspirant device, *J. Clin. Eng.,* 8(3), 253, 1983.

31. Rosengren, L., Bäcklund, Y., Sjöström, T., Kök, B., and Svedbergh, B., A system for wireless intra-ocular pressure measurements using a silicon micromachined sensor, *J. Micromach. Microeng.,* 2, 202, 1992.

32. Wouters, P., De Cooman, M., Lapadatu, D., and Puers, R., A low power multi-sensor interface for injectable microprocessor-based animal monitoring system, *Sensors Actuators A,* 41–42, 198, 1994.

33. Park, J., Choi, S., Heedon, S., and Nakamura, T., Fabrication of CMOS IC for telemetering biological signals from multiple subjects, *Sensors Actuators A,* 43, 289, 1994.

7 Iontophoresis of Peptides

M. Begoña Delgado-Charro
and Richard H. Guy

CONTENTS

7.1 INTEREST AND RATIONALE

The advantages of transdermal drug administration have been well documented, and many passive delivery systems have been developed. However, the excellent barrier function of the skin, and the lipophilic nature of the stratum corneum in particular, means that the useful transport of charged and/or highly polar drugs requires an effective enhancement strategy.

Iontophoresis, of course, represents one such approach and its application to the delivery of pharmacologically active peptides has attracted significant attention (see Table 7.1). In addition to their inherent interest, peptides serve as models for other classes of new biotechnology drugs, such as small proteins and oligonucleotides. The succesful systemic delivery of these compounds poses a very real problem to the pharmaceutical scientist. Chronic intravenous or intramuscular administration is clearly undesirable. Oral dosing presents major stability and absorption difficulties. Other potential routes (e.g., implants, rectal, nasal) suffer from different, but equally significant, problems. The objectives of this chapter, therefore, are to review the

0-8493-7681-5/98/$0.00+$.50
© 1998 by CRC Press LLC

TABLE 7.1

Summary of Research Involving the Study of Peptide Delivery by Iontophoresis

Compound	Model	Technique	Variables measured	Ref.
Amino acids	Hairless mouse	*In vitro* diffusion cells	Iontophoretic flux	1
Amino acids	Hairless rat	*In vitro* diffusion cells	Iontophoretic flux, binding	2
Amino acids and N-acetyl derivatives	Hairless mouse	*In vitro* diffusion cells	Iontophoretic flux	3
Tripeptides Ac-Ala-X-Ala-NH (Bu^t)	Hairless mouse	*In vitro* diffusion cells	Iontophoretic flux	4
Threo-Lys-Pro	Nude rat	*In vitro* diffusion cells, *in vivo* iontophoresis	*In vitro* iontophoretic flux, *in vivo* distribution in the skin, cumulative urinary excretion	5
TRH	Nude mouse	*In vitro* diffusion cells	Iontophoretic flux	6
	Hairless rat	*In vitro* diffusion cells	TRH distribution and localization in the skin	7
TRH and desamino-tyrosyl lysil prolineamide		*In vitro* diffusion cells	Iontophoretic flux	8
TRH	Human cadaver	*In vitro* diffusion cells	Iontophoretic flux	9
Enalaprilat	Hairless guinea pig	*In vitro* diffusion cells	Iontophoretic flux	10
Angiotensin	Hairless mouse	*In vitro* diffusion cells	Iontophoretic flux	11
Octreotide	Rabbits	*In vivo* iontophoresis	AUC; C_{max}; t_{max}	12
GRF analog	Hairless guinea pig	*In vitro* diffusion cells	Iontophoretic flux	13
		In vivo iontophoresis	Plasma levels; half-life; AUC; volume distribution	14
AVP	Hairless rat	*In vitro* diffusion cells	Iontophoretic flux	15
		In vitro diffusion cells	Iontophoretic flux	16
		In vitro diffusion cells	Iontophoretic flux	17
	Human cadaver	*In vitro* diffusion cell	Iontophoretic flux, metabolism	18
1-Desamino-8-D-arginine vasopressin	Human cadaver	*In vitro* diffusion cells	Iontophoretic flux	19
AVP and 1-desamino-8-D-arginine vasopressin	Wistar rat	*In vivo* iontophoresis	Antidiuretic effect, metabolism inhibitors	20
		In vivo iontophoresis	Antidiuretic effect	21
9-Desglycinamide, 8-arginine-vasopressin	Human (surgery)	*In vitro* diffusion cells	Iontophoretic flux	22
	Human stratum corneum and shed snake	*In vitro* diffusion cells	Iontophoretic flux	23
Salmon calcitonin	Wistar rat	*In vivo* iontophoresis	Plasma calcium levels, metabolism inhibitors	24
	Hairless guinea pig Testskin™	*In vitro* diffusion cells	Iontophoretic flux	25, 56

TABLE 7.1 (continued)
Summary of Research Involving the Study of Peptide Delivery by Iontophoresis

Compound	Model	Technique	Variables measured	Ref.
Human calcitonin	Hairless rat	*In vitro* diffusion cells *In vivo* iontophoresis	*In vitro* iontophoretic flux, plasma calcium levels	26
		In vitro iontophoresis	*In vitro* iontophoretic flux	17
LHRH and [DTrp⁶, Pro⁹-NHEt]LHRH	Hairless mouse	*In vitro* iontophoresis	*In vitro* iontophoretic flux	27
LHRH	Yorkshire pigs	IPPSF iontophoresis *In vivo* iontophoresis	IPPSF iontophoretic flux *In vivo* LHRH, LH, and FSH plasma levels	28
LHRH	Yorkshire pigs	IPPSF repeated iontophoresis	Iontophoretic flux	29
	Human cadaver	*In vitro* diffusion cells	Iontophoretic flux, electroporative flux	30
	Hairless rat	*In vitro* diffusion cells	Iontophoretic flux	31
Buserelin	Human stratum corneum	*In vitro* rotating disk cells	Iontophoretic flux	32
Nafarelin	Hairless mouse	*In vitro* diffusion cells	Iontophoretic flux	33, 34
	Human cadaver	*In vitro* diffusion cells	Iontophoretic flux	35
Leuprolide	Human	*In vitro* diffusion cells	Iontophoretic flux	36
	Human epidermis Nucleopore™	*In vitro* diffusion cells	Iontophoretic flux	37
	Human	*In vivo* iontophoresis	Serum LH and testosterone	38, 39
		In vivo iontophoresis	Serum leuprolide, LH, and testosterone	40
Cholecystokinin-8	Human	*In vitro* diffusion cell	Iontophoretic flux	36
Methionine enkephalin	Hairless mouse	*In vitro* diffusion cell	Iontophoretic flux	41
Porcine insulin	Hairless rat	*In vitro* diffusion cell	Iontophoretic flux	17
		In vitro diffusion cell	Iontophoretic flux	42
	Human surgery	*In vitro* diffusion cell	Iontophoretic flux	43
Monomeric insulin analogs	Hairless mouse	*In vitro* diffusion cell	Iontophoretic flux	44, 45
Insulin	Hairless rat	*In vitro* diffusion cell *In vivo* iontophoresis	*In vitro* iontophoretic flux Glycemia	46
	Human, swine	*In vivo* iontophoresis	Glucose and insulin plasma levels	47
Human insulin	Rabbits	*In vivo* iontophoresis	Glucose and insulin plasma levels	48
Insulin	Human	*In vivo* iontophoresis	Sweat [Cl⁻]	49
	Rabbits	*In vivo* iontophoresis	Glucose and insulin plasma levels	50
	Hairless rat, rabbits	*In vivo* iontophoresis	Glucose and insulin plasma levels	51–55
Bovine serum albumin	Hairless mouse	*In vitro* diffusion cell	Iontophoretic flux	1

current state of the art in peptide iontophoresis, to examine the mechanistic implications of the results obtained, and to identify the key experimental and formulation
variables that impact upon the efficiency of peptide delivery.

7.2 MECHANISMS

Iontophoresis enhances the transdermal delivery of substances by three different
mechanisms: electrorepulsion, electro-osmosis, and electrically induced skin permeability changes. These three mechanisms are operative for iontophoresis of peptides,
and their relative importance has been studied. With an alternative electrical enhancement technique, namely, electroporation, the transport observed is higher than with
iontophoresis. The mechanisms of iontophoresis and electroporation appear to be
completely different: whereas in iontophoresis the flux is related to the total charge
transported through the system, electroporative voltage pulses produce transient
permeabilization of the stratum corneum and transport cannot be related to the
amount of charge passed across the skin.[30] In this chapter, discussion is limited
specifically to iontophoresis.

7.2.1 ELECTROREPULSION

Electrorepulsion is the result of the direct interaction of molecules with the applied
field. According to Faraday's law:

$$J_a^T = \frac{t_a^T I}{Z_a F} = \frac{Z_a U_a C_a^T}{\sum\limits_{i=1}^{n} z_i U_i C_i^T} \left(\frac{I}{Z_a F} \right) = \frac{I U_a C_a^T}{F \sum\limits_{i=1}^{n} z_i U_i C_i^T}$$

the iontophoretic flux of compound "a" at time $T(J_a^T)$ is related to the applied current
(I), to the compound transport number (t_a^T), electrical mobility (u_a), charge (Z_a),
concentration (c_a) and to the concentrations, mobilities and charges of the other ions
present in the system (c_i, u_i, z_i).

It follows that, if all the other factors remain constant, then the transdermal flux
of ion "a" should be controllable by modulating the applied current density. This
feature of iontophoresis constitutes its main attraction, in that it offers the opportunity
to adapt the delivery input rate to the particularities of each patient or phase of the
treatment. In this way, the development of an externally controlled delivery system
can be envisaged. Such a possibility would be particularly interesting for certain
peptides such as luteinizing hormone–releasing hormone (LHRH) analogs which
have different pharmacological effects depending on their delivery-input rate,[57] vasopressin, for which pulsatile delivery is preferred to avoid downregulation and tolerance,[18] or GRF (growth hormone–releasing factor) for which delivery only at night
is preferred.[14]

Iontophoresis has been performed at either constant voltage or constant current.
Faraday's and Ohm's laws clearly indicate, however, that constant current controls
flux most efficiently and reliably. Indeed, constant voltage iontophoresis of peptides

has been much less frequently reported.[13,14,24,36,37,43] The literature is completely consistent on the fact that the imposition of an electrical field across the skin causes the resistance of the barrier to decrease. This fall in resistance is more marked at higher applied voltages or currents.[58,59] This observation together with Ohm's law ($V = IR$) shows clearly why constant current iontophoresis is the only *sensible* approach when developing a controllable drug delivery system. At constant voltage, a fall in R requires current to increase in order that Ohm's law be satisfied; then, however, according to Faraday's law, the flux of the ion of interest will change, and it will change according to a noncontrolled parameter, that is, the skin resistance. At constant current, on the other hand, a decrease in R merely provokes a decrease in applied voltage to meet the demands of Ohm's law. The total charge flowing across the skin, though, and hence the ion fluxes, remain controlled by the current. The undeniable logic of the above arguments is supported by the literature. For example, when constant voltage iontophoresis of a GRF analog (Ro 23-7861) was performed,[13] the flux correlated better with the resultant current that was produced under the different experimental conditions employed than with the voltage. This decisive role of current density as the delivery-controlling factor was confirmed *in vivo*: it was found that, to maintain control of drug input, the iontophoretic device had to be modified to incorporate a maximum limiting current.[14]

The total charge delivered in iontophoresis can be increased by using a higher current density i.e., keeping area constant and passing a higher current, by maintaining current density constant and increasing surface area, or by a longer application time. If all effects are linear, these factors should be interchangeable. There is good evidence that the iontophoretic flux of small peptides (e.g., TRH[6] and the tripeptide Threo-Lys-Pro[5]) increases with current density *in vitro*. For these small tripeptides, linear correlations between flux and current density have been observed. For larger peptides, however, the results are more divergent. While angiotensin iontophoresis flux increased quite linearly with current density[11] (Figure 7.1), for DGAVP (9-desglycinamide, 8-arginine-vasopressin) a poor correlation was observed between flux and current;[22] in fact, a more than sixfold increment in current density did not even double the flux. AVP (arginine-vasopressin) enhancement factors increased with current density applied either periodically or continuously.[16] In this case, though, application time and current density were not interchangeable factors; keeping the total charge delivered constant, more peptide transport was observed for higher currents (short application times) than for lower (longer application times). *In vivo*, the antidiuretic response of AVP and its analog 1-deamino-8-D-arginine vasopressin (1-d-8-DAVP)[21] increased with increasing total charge applied (either by increasing current density or by prolonging the duration of iontophoresis). Also, the bioavailability of octreotide in rabbits increased directly with the applied current.[12] On the other hand, for calcitonin, increasing the period of iontophoresis did not enhance the *in vitro* flux, and increasing the total charge delivered did not cause a significantly greater decrease in calcaemia *in vivo* in rats.[26]

The linear relationship between LHRH flux and current density was restricted to the lower values of current (<1.25 mA/cm^2) considered;[30] at higher currents, peptide transport correlated better with i^2, suggesting that flux was proportional to the energy delivered. Electroheating was suggested as a possible mechanism to

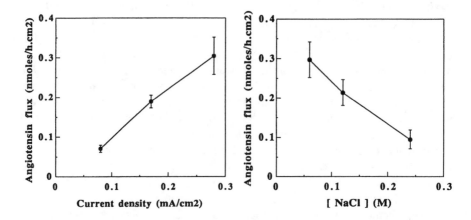

FIGURE 7.1 Iontophoretic flux of angiotensin through hairless mouse skin *in vitro* as a function of (a) current density and (b) electrolyte concentration. The concentration of angiotensin in the donor anode chamber (pH = 6.5) was 95.6 nmol/mL; current was passed for a period of up to 5 h. The data shown are mean ± SD (*n* = 6). (Results redrawn from Reference 11.)

explain these results. The issue may be moot, however, as it is generally accepted that the maximum current density tolerable for therapeutic purposes is ≤0.5 mA/cm².[60]

LHRH analogs have shown significant deviations from the anticipated behavior. The flux of the analog D-[Trp⁶,Pro⁹-NHEt] LHRH showed only a twofold increase when the current was increased by a factor of five (Figure 7.2).[27] Iontophoresis of leuprolide through human skin was initially reported to be unsuccessful without ethanol pretreatment;[36] later work from the same group, again with leuprolide,[37] and from our own research using nafarelin[33-35,61] (both in human and hairless mouse skin) revealed that the electrorepulsive contribution to the iontophoretic flux was overwhelmed by the ability of the peptides to alter the skin permselectivity and the direction of the electro-osmotic flow (Figure 7.3) (see below). Transport followed, therefore, a highly unexpected dependence upon current density. Nevertheless, despite these complicated behaviors, the successful iontophoresis of leuprolide "*in vivo*" in humans, at very low current density (0.2 mA applied over 70 cm²) has been reported.[38,39]

Overall, the data suggest that iontophoretic peptide flux correlates reasonably well with current in the practical range, but that some important deviations have been observed. Exceptions generally correspond to situations in which electrorepulsion is no longer the major mechanism of electrotransport and for which electro-osmosis is the crucial phenomenon (see below).

Both pulsed and continuous direct current have been used, whereas alternating current has seldom been applied for peptides.[41] The rationale for pulsed current application is twofold. In a "macroscopic" sense, the principal objective is to generate a peptide input rate that mimics the physiological pattern of, for example, hormonal release; indeed, pulsatile iontophoretic delivery has been demonstrated for several peptides.[16,27,32] In this application of pulsatile current passage, the "on" and "off" periods of charge delivery are measured in times on the order of minutes. In the second, "microscope", manifestation of pulsed current application, several authors

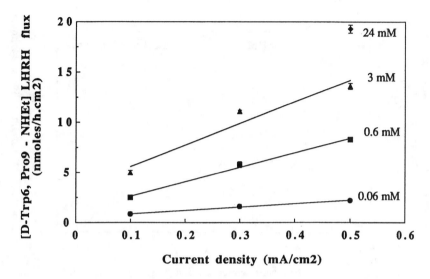

FIGURE 7.2 The effects of varying current density and peptide concentration on the iontophoretic flux of [D-Trp^6,Pro^9-NHEt]LHRH across hairless mouse skin *in vitro*. The background electrolyte in the donor solution was an unspecified concentration of sodium chloride; the pH was not reported. Current was passed for 5 h. The data shown are mean ± SD ($n =$ 4). (Results redrawn from Reference 27.)

have claimed various advantages for the use of rapid "on–off" protocols (measured now in times of fractions of seconds) over continuous current.[53]

A number of studies have compared pulsed and continuous direct current, and have also explored the effect of frequency and duty cycle.[11,13,15,16,22,26,32,46] For example, for angiotensin,[11] the direct current iontophoretic flux at 0.28 mA/cm^2, pH 6.5, was 0.226 ± 0.04 nmol/h·cm^2, a value approximately double that when a pulsed current profile (on–off ratio 1:1, frequency 100 Hz) was used (0.100 ± 0.019 nmol/h·cm^2). This result is, of course, consistent with the efficiency of delivery being proportional to the on period of current application. However, in the same article, when the effect of pulsed frequency was examined, two inconsistent observations were reported: first, a replicate experiment at 1000 Hz and the same current density resulted in a significantly smaller peptide flux (0.043 ± 0.011 nmol/h·cm^2); second, as the frequency was increased from 0.5 to 15 KHz, angiotensin flux increased approximately 2.2-fold (0.041 ± 0.017 to 0.091 ± 0.024 nmol/h·cm^2). [*Note*: the authors incorrectly report this change as 3.5-fold, and the significance of the differences between the fluxes measured at different frequencies is not reported.]

For DGAVP[22] there was no effect of duty cycle (25 to 99%) or frequency (10 Hz to 10 kHz) on the steady-state flux when the mean current density was kept constant. For AVP[16] "pulsed-continuous" iontophoresis was more successful than "pulsed-periodically" applied current, even after correcting the values for different times.*

---

* "Pulsed-continuous" current with square-waveform was applied at a frequency of 2 kHz with an on–off ratio of 1:1. For "pulsed-periodic" current application, one cycle comprised "pulsed current" on (frequency 2 kHz, on–off ratio 1:1) for 10 min and current off for 30 min.

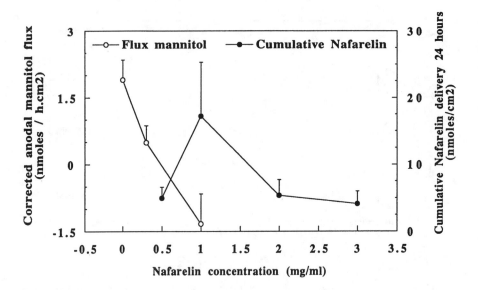

FIGURE 7.3 Comparison between cumulative nafarelin delivery by iontophoresis across hairless mouse skin *in vitro*, with the concomitant electro-osmotic flow (as measured by the transport of the uncharged, nonmetabolizable sugar mannitol), as a function of the initial nafarelin concentration in the donor anode chamber. The current density was 0.63 mA/cm^2 passed for 24 h in the case of nafarelin, and 0.55 mA/cm^2 passed for 12 h for mannitol. The supporting electrolyte was 14 mM NaCl for nafarelin and 0.17 M phosphate buffer containing 44 mM NaCl, pH 7.4 for mannitol. Data are shown as mean ± SD ($n = 3$ to 6). (Results redrawn from References 34 and 61.)

For this peptide a reproducible pulsatile delivery was achieved, although steady state was not attained for the higher currents; there was no effect of frequency (0 to 16 KHz).

No differences in calcitonin flux *in vitro* were found between pulsed and continuous treatments at the same mean current density. However, *in vivo*, pulsed current produced significantly prolonged effects on calcaemia (i.e., lowering of calcium blood levels) than continuous current.[26]

GRF[13] fluxes at frequencies ranging from 40 to 50 KHz were not significantly different when a constant voltage device was used; but the measured current and the total amount of peptide delivered increased slightly with increasing frequency.

Blood glucose levels in diabetic rats were not affected by the iontophoretic administration of insulin using constant current; they were, however, reduced by pulsed current.[51] The effects were dependent on frequency, waveform, and duty cycle. A minimum frequency of 1 kHz was necessary to achieve a significant lowering of glucose levels, and the reduction was more marked at higher frequencies. The optimum on–off ratio was 1:1. *In vitro*, insulin iontophoretic fluxes were also higher for pulsed than for continuous current.[46] According to the authors of this work, the beneficial effects of pulsatile current result from the reduced polarization of the skin which occurs with continuous current.[51]

The contradictory results observed with pulsed and continuous iontophoresis of peptides may be complicated by binding, accumulation, and altered electro-osmotic flow. As discussed below, this certainly appears to be the case with nafarelin.[33] Significant binding of calcitonin has also been reported,[26] leading to the apparent establishment of a reservoir from which the peptide can slowly diffuse after termination of current flow. For example, a constant flux has been observed for 7 h even though current had been applied for only 60 min. In the case of appreciable accumulation of peptide in the skin, it is conceivable that modulation of current flow (periodicity or sign, for example) might be used to optimize the delivery of the drug.

7.2.2 Convective Flow

At physiological pH, the skin supports a net negative charge and is therefore permselective to cations; this characteristic provides the basis for a second mechanism of electrotransport.[62] For a negatively charged membrane, the counterions (i.e., cations) are preferentially attracted into the barrier. In moving under the influence of the applied field, the ions collide with the surrounding solvent molecules and transfer a fraction of their momentum. In the case of the skin, with its net negative charge, more momentum is, therefore, transferred in the direction of the counterion flow. Thus, there is an electro-osmotic flow of water across the skin during iontophoresis in the anode-to-cathode direction. Furthermore, it follows that uncharged solutes dissolved in the solvent will also be convected with the solvent flow across the skin in the same direction.

Thus, electro-osmotic flow allows the delivery of neutral compounds and assists in the delivery of cationic solutes. For example, the normalized anodic iontophoretic flux of zwitterionic amino acids and tripeptides is higher than the cathodic flux, and the flux of cationic species is greater than that of similar size anions; these results show the preferential direction of the convective flow under normal physiological conditions.[3,4,63] Convective transport of the neutral solute mannitol is dependent on the current density, pH, and ionic strength and concentration.[61,62,64-66] To some extent, convective transport is size independent, so its relative contribution to electrotransport increases with the molecular weight of the solute.[62]

The relative contributions of electrorepulsion and electro-osmosis to the total transport of a particular compound have been inferred but not quantitatively determined. Experimental conditions such as solute concentration, current density, ionic strength, pH, etc., have different but simultaneous effects on electrorepulsion and electro-osmosis that are difficult to separate. Nevertheless, there is general agreement that convection assumes a more important role as the size of the transported solute increases. Most peptides are large relative to the ubiquituosly present and much more mobile ions of the electrolyte, such as sodium or chloride; thus, transport numbers for peptides are invariably very low, e.g., 3×10^{-3} for angiotensin;[11] 4.5×10^{-6} for LHRH;[30] 6.7×10^{-4} for TRH;[6] 10^{-5} for Thr-Lys-Pro.[5] Hence, there is support for the hypothesis that electro-osmosis plays a decisive role in peptide iontophoresis. Furthermore, for very large negative solutes, it has been proposed (and for which there is a small amount of experimental support) that increased electrotransport is achievable, and is likely to be more efficient, by "wrong-way" iontophoresis; in other words, electro-osmosis from the anode offers the most likely approach to achieve measurable delivery.[1,6] However, the efficiency of this approach is necessarily very small indeed.

The first approach to quantify the role of convection in peptide iontophoresis was to analyze the impact of changing the pH on the flux.[3,4] Lysine, for example, is a cationic amino acid (relevant $pK_a > 10$), which is essentially fully positively charged at pH 7.4, and is very efficiently iontophoresed under these conditions. Lowering the pH to 4 leads to a reduction in flux, presumably due to some neutralization of the net negative charge on the skin and a loss of the electro-osmotic contribution to electrotransport. Histidine, on the other hand, which is also capable of carrying a net charge of +1, has the relevant pK_a at 6. Thus, the neutral form predominates at pH 7 while the cation is principally present at pH 4. In this case, the dominant effect of electrorepulsion means that the flux is higher at the lower pH. The same is true for the tripeptide Ac-Ala-His-Ala-NH(Bu^t). A different peptide, namely, TRH,[6] shows different behavior in that its iontophoretic flux is greater at pH 8 (where the peptide is neutral) than at pH 4 (where it is charged). The transport number of TRH was found to be very low under the conditions at which its electrotransport was studied, an observation consistent with the more important role of electro-osmosis in this example. Unfortunately, as with much of the literature on peptide iontophoresis, direct comparison of the behavior of different compounds is difficult because of the different conditions used (pH, ionic strength, current density, animal model, etc.). It is clear that the pH values on either side of the skin "*in vitro*" can have profound effects on electro-osmosis.

Angiotensin flux changed only slightly when the pH of the donor solution was increased from 6.5 to 8.5, despite the fact that the peptide is uncharged at the higher pH.[11] Lowering the pH from 6.5 to 4.5 provoked a quite dramatic reduction in flux. A similar effect on peptide flux was observed when calcium ions were used instead of sodium in the background electrolyte donor solution. Likewise, the transport of water with and without calcium ions showed parallel behavior. These results support a significant contribution of convection to the electrotransport of angiotensin. Nevertheless, it appears that electrorepulsion is still important: an increment of current density, that caused a 1.6-fold increase in the transport of water, resulted in a fourfold increase in the transport of angiotensin.

For DGAVP[22] the data also support the hypothesis that both electrorepulsive and electro-osmotic mechanisms are operative. Anodic delivery increases with pH (from 5 to 7.4) due presumably to the increase in convection. At pH 8, which corresponds to the pI of the peptide, flux is smaller than at pH 7.4 and pH 6 but higher than that at pH 3 and 5. At both pH 5 and at the pI, reducing the ionic strength by a factor of ten caused flux to increase fivefold. Obviously, at pH 8 this effect is due not to the change in ionic competition but to the effect of ionic strength on electro-osmosis.[62,65]

In conclusion, the published data show that, for amino acids such as histidine and lysine (155 and 146 MW), an important contribution of electrorepulsion exists. For larger tripeptides (e.g., thyrotropin, 363 MW, and Ala-His-Ala, 394 MW) and certainly octa-, nona-, and decapeptides (angiotensin, 1046; DGAVP, 1080, nafarelin,

1321 MW) the contribution of electro-osmosis becomes progressively more important. The extreme (i.e., complete dominance by electro-osmosis) is represented by the anodic, wrong-way iontophoresis of large anionic compounds (bovine serum albumin, 69000 MW) and carboxyinulin (5200 MW) at pH 8.6.[1]

Wrong-way iontophoresis represents a situation equivalent to that in capillary zone electrophoresis (CZE) in which the fraction of surface silanols carrying a negative charge depends on the pH. In CZE, conditions are set up to achieve significant electro-osmosis so that all analytes eventually migrate with the solvent flow regardless of the electric charge.[67] Whether or not a CZE-equivalent situation is possible in transdermal iontophoresis of peptides remains unproven. While the idea is supported by some results for carboxyinulin,[1] data for salmon calcitonin are less clear. The pI of this peptide is 6.5,[24] and it has been administered by iontophoresis to rats *in vivo*. No effects on plasma calcium levels were observed when the anodic donor solution was either at pH 5.5, pH 7, or pH 8 (peptide +; –; –); however, there was an effect with the donor solution at pH 4. It should be noted, though, that in these experiments the receptor phase pH is fixed at physiological; it has been demonstrated that hairless mouse skin retains cation permselectivity when the donor (anode) solution is at pH 4 and the receptor at pH 7.4. Overall, then, it appears that wrong-way iontophoresis of this peptide is not possible.

An important demonstration of the decisive role that electro-osmosis can play in the iontophoretic delivery of peptides is provided by the analogs of LHRH. Many of these analogs involve substitution of the amino acid at position 6 (glycine) in LHRH[57] with a more lipophilic moiety. A relationship between lipophilicity and peptide potency has been observed.[57] Following iontophoresis, an important depot in the skin is established for LHRH[29] and nafarelin.[33] Aside from issues pertaining to reservoir effects, delivery rate, dosing, etc., the accumulation of lipophilic LHRH analogs produces unexpected effects on the permselective properties of the barrier. The binding of these lipophilic, cationic compounds to the skin appears to neutralize the negative charge on the membrane, and to change thereby the direction of electro-osmotic flow (Figure 7.3). The iontophoretic flux of mannitol, a neutral marker, is preferentially from anode to cathode under normal physiological circumstances (i.e., donor and receptor chamber at pH 7.4).[66] When a lipophilic LHRH analog (e.g., nafarelin or leuprolide) is anodically iontophoresed in the presence of mannitol, a highly significant decrease in electro-osmotic flow (i.e., in the flux of the neutral sugar) is observed.[33,34,37,61] If side-by-side diffusion cells are used, it is possible to show, when the peptide is present in the anodal chamber,[33,37] that not only is the electro-osmotic cotransport of the neutral compound from the anodal solution decreased, but also that the reverse electro-osmosis is increased. This is entirely consistent with the net charge on the membrane changing from negative to positive. The effect is particularly significant for leuprolide[37] and nafarelin,[33,34,61] but to a much smaller extent for the less hydrophobic LHRH.[61] The magnitude of the effect on convective flow is correlated with peptide concentration and the current density applied.[34,61] The lipophilicity of the peptide is important because if, instead of nafarelin, the mixture of cationic amino acids present in the peptide is anodally iontophoresed, there is *no* effect on the convective flow.[61] Overall, these results suggest that large, lipophilic and cationic species are necessary to evoke the dramatic changes in electro-osmotic flow. However, more recently, Hirvonen et al.[68-70] have shown that lipophilic cationic tripeptides (e.g., D-naphthylalanine-leucine-arginine, the 6 to 8 residues of nafarelin) and even certain simpler, lipophilic and positively chargeable drugs (e.g., propranolol) can induce the same effects on convective solvent movement as the larger peptides. The phenomenon may be likened to the reversal of electro-osmosis in capillary electrophoresis due to the adsorption of cationic surfactants onto the capillary walls[71] (indeed, nafarelin does itself have certain tensioactive properties[72]).

The consequences of this behavior on iontophoretic peptide delivery are self-evident, in particular that the flux of the peptide, and of any other solute transported by electro-osmosis, is seriously perturbed. The magnitude, by which the flux of a molecule is decreased, depends directly on the relative contribution of electro-osmosis to the total flux. For peptides, in addition to the LHRH analogs, such as nafarelin and leuprolide, there is evidence that this mechanism also impacts upon the delivery of octreotide[12] and calcitonin.[26]

This phenomenon explains several experimental results that have been obtained with different peptides. In particular, there are several examples in which either a nonlinear, or even inverse, correlation between peptide iontophoretic flux and concentration or current density has been observed (e.g., nafarelin, leuprolide, D-Trp[6]-LHRH, octreotide, and calcitonin). As the current density or concentration is increased, more peptide is transported into, and accumulated in, the skin, causing the net negative charge on the membrane to decrease. This leads to inhibition of electro-osmosis and a consequent reduction in peptide transport. For human calcitonin in hairless rat skin, for example, neither the flux nor the cumulative amount of peptide delivered increased with longer periods of current passage.[26]

There is also evidence of the critical role of electro-osmosis in peptide iontophoresis in humans. The steady-state concentrations of leuprolide, for example, and the area under the plasma concentration vs. time curve decreased as the peptide concentration in the iontophoretic patch was increased[40] (Figure 7.4). Conversely, in another study with the same peptide,[38,39] the use of extremely low current density (3.1 μA/cm^2), a large surface area (70 cm^2), and a smaller applied concentration (5 mg/mL) elicit a pharmacologically meaningful effect on *in vivo* LH (luteinizing hormone) levels in human subjects. This latter finding suggests that the experimental conditions used provoked a much less important perturbation of electro-osmosis and correspondingly, a much smaller inhibition of peptide flux.

In another example (Figure 7.5), it was found that the bioavailability of iontophoretically delivered octreotide in rabbits decreased with increasing peptide concentration,[12] but increased with current density (in the range 50 to 150 μA/cm^2).

Ignoring any size restrictions, the convective transport of a molecule is expected to be proportional to its concentration in the solvent;[62] i.e., doubling the concentration of a peptide, which is iontophoretically moved across the skin by electro-osmosis, should double the amount absorbed.

Thus, the fact that this does not occur for all peptides lends support to the argument that some compounds are capable of altering the net charge of the skin, and hence the permselectivity of (and electro-osmotic flow through) the membrane. It is also true that, at fixed peptide concentration, increasing the iontophoretic current

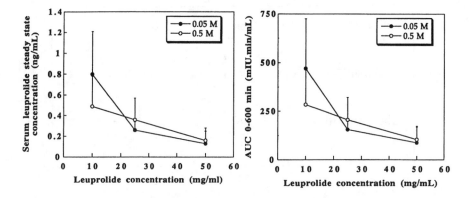

FIGURE 7.4 Iontophoretic delivery of leuprolide *in vivo*, in humans, as a function of peptide concentration and of the ionic strength of the background electrolyte in the donor anode chamber. Current (0.2 mA) was applied over an unspecified area of skin. Data shown represent the mean ± SD (*n* = 5 to 6). (Results redrawn from Reference 40.)

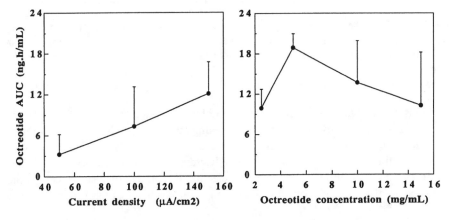

FIGURE 7.5 Iontophoretic delivery of octreotide *in vivo*, in rabbits, as a function of current density ([peptide] = 5 mg/mL) and peptide concentration (current density = 150 µA/cm²) in the donor anode chamber. Current was passed for 6 and 8 h, respectively. The background electrolyte was 100 mM NaCl. Data shown represent mean ± SD (*n* = 3 to 4). (Results redrawn from Reference 12.)

will (1) provoke more electro-osmosis, but (2) drive more peptide into the skin (which will, in turn, for peptides like leuprolide and nafarelin, for example, cause convective flow to be reduced). Although these two effects operate in competition, the experimental evidence supports dominance of the former, i.e., the increased current causes a greater increase in electro-osmosis than the reduction induced by the elevated amount of peptide in the skin (Figure 7.6). This appears to be the situation for nafarelin and octreotide. For these peptides, at fixed current density, increased donor concentration leads to decreased flux; conversely, at fixed concentration,

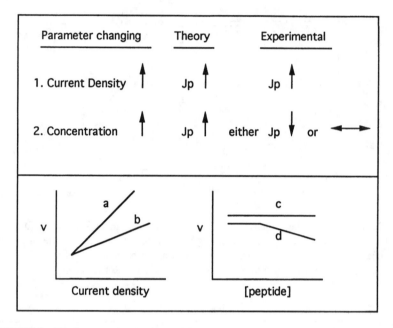

FIGURE 7.6   The impact of cationic peptide alteration of skin permselectivity on (1) [upper panel] peptide flux (J_p), and (2) [lower panel] electro-osmotic flow (v), as a function of current density and peptide concentration. In the lower panel, curves a and c illustrate typical results for a peptide that does not associate with the skin, while curves b and d schematically show the pattern of behavior observed for a peptide which significantly changes skin permselectivity.

increasing the current density increased the flux, although the enhancement is not fully linear (a fact consistent with the competing effects of a higher current). It might be suggested that the concentration and current dependencies of compounds such as nafarelin might be diagnostic of two factors: (1) that electro-osmosis is the principal mechanism of enhancement by electrotransport and (2) that the compound is capable of altering the overall charge and permselectivity of the skin.

7.2.3   Current-Induced Permeability Changes

The majority of peptide iontophoresis studies (indeed, of all iontophoretic experiments) have been conducted *in vitro*. It is generally the case that the post-iontophoretic passive permeability of the skin is greater than the pretreatment value. Thus, it is clear that current passage *in vitro* causes skin barrier function to change. However, at the present time, there is very little information on the extent to which this phenomenon is manifest *in vivo*. While it is known that rapid and substantial changes in skin impedance occur with current passage, little or no change in transepidermal water loss (a typical marker of the passive diffusion barrier of the skin) is induced.[59,73] Obviously, *in vitro*, the skin cannot completely recover from any applied perturbation and its overall viability will continue to diminish with time. Hence, it is unwise, in our opinion, to extrapolate *in vitro* current-induced permeability changes to the *in vivo* situation.

From the limited *in vivo* data available, it is known the current passage can be used to increase the passive permeability of hairless rat skin to a tripeptide (Thr-Lys-Pro).[5] Importantly, despite the comments above, good coincidence with *in vitro* results was found in this case. In the isolated perfused porcine skin flap (IPPSF), an *"ex vivo"* model that maintains skin viability more closely to that *in vivo* than any other, it has also been shown that a second period of iontophoresis delivered more peptide (in this case, LHRH) than the first, when the electrodes were placed at the same skin sites.[29] If different sites were used for the second iontophoretic period, however, the delivery was not statistically different from that during the first. It should be emphasized that many open questions remain, not the least of which relate to whether the permselective properties of the membrane are constant, whether biochemical (metabolic) capabilities have been altered, whether the pH profile across the barrier is the same, etc.

An important potential advantage of peptide iontophoresis is the ability to achieve pulsatile drug input. This means that the flux achieves a target value quickly after current initiation, then falls to zero when the current is turned off, only to regain the target level on reconnection of the current, etc. *In vitro*, this desired pattern has been achieved for a number of peptides, including AVP,[16,19] LHRH analogs [D-Trp^6,Pro^9-NHEt]LHRH[27] and buserelin ([D-Ser(Bu^t)^6,Pro^9-NHEt]LHRH).[32] In the latter case, however, at higher current densities, the flux increased with reapplication of the current. For other peptides (e.g., certain tripeptides,[4] calcitonin,[26] and LHRH[30]), conversely, post-iontophoresis transport is clearly elevated over the pre-current levels. There is, furthermore, a problem associated with the flux falling quickly to zero on current termination for peptides that form any sort of reservoir in the skin — nafarelin is an example of such a compound. In this situation, experience teaches that the most practical realization of an *in vivo* device may involve delivery of the compound at low current density over as large a skin surface area as possible.

7.3 FACTORS DETERMINING PEPTIDE IONTOPHORETIC FLUX

7.3.1 PHYSICOCHEMICAL CHARACTERISTICS: SIZE, LIPOPHILICITY, AND CHARGE

It should be stated at the outset that direct comparison of the iontophoretic fluxes of different peptides, as a function of one or more physicochemical factors, is very difficult owing to the wide variety of experimental conditions used (e.g., pH, ionic strength, buffer composition, electrodes, skin source, etc.). To provide some idea of the range of results reported in the literature, we have collected together in Table 7.2, the normalized fluxes (i.e., flux at time t hours postinitiation of anodal iontophoresis divided by applied concentration divided by current density) of various peptides and other compounds; these data were obtained from experiments in which the donor and receptor solutions were maintained at pH values between 6 and 8. The molecular weights of the delivered compounds are also given in the table.

TABLE 7.2
Values of Normalized Flux (NF) for Various Peptides and for Selected Uncharged Markers

Compound	M.W.	Current mA·cm⁻²	Conc. (C) μmol·cm⁻³	Flux (J) nmol·h⁻¹·cm⁻²	10⁹·J/C m·sec⁻¹	Skin[g]	10⁹·N F m³·sec⁻¹·A⁻¹	Ref.
Glycine	75[a]	0.32	50.0	6.0[d]	16.7	HMS	5.21	1
Alanine	89[a]	0.36	10.0	10.0	2.79	HMS	0.77	3
Lysine	146[c]	0.36	10.0	131	36.4	HMS	11.1	3
Glucose	180[a]	0.32	50.0	4.0[d]	11.1	HMS	3.47	1
Tyrosine	181[b]	0.32	2.0	2.0[d]	6.49	HMS	2.17	1
Mannitol	182[a]	0.55	1.0	0.81	2.25	HMS	0.41	61
	182[a]	0.42	1.0	0.80	2.22	HMS	0.53	61
Lactose	360[a]	0.42	1.0	1.18	3.28	HMS	0.78	61
Sucrose	342[a]	0.55	1.0	0.89	2.47	HMS	0.45	61
Thr-Lys-Pro	344[c]	0.18	1.0	0.12	0.33	NuRat	0.18	5
	344[c]	0.27	1.0	0.19	0.53	NuRat	0.19	5
	344[c]	0.36	1.0	0.27	0.75	NuRat	0.21	5
TRH	362[a]	0.16	8.8	11.2	3.55	NuMS	2.22	6
	362[a]	0.31	8.8	23.7	7.50	NuMS	2.42	6
	362[a]	0.47	8.8	32.5	10.3	NuMS	2.18	6
Angiotensin	1046[c]	0.28[e]	0.09	0.23	6.57	HMS	2.35	11
	1046[c]	0.28[f]	0.09	0.09	2.62	HMS	0.93	11
	1046[c]	0.17	0.09	0.18	5.23	HMS	3.08	11
	1046[c]	0.08	0.09	0.08	2.32	HMS	2.91	11
DGAVP	1080[c]	0.13	1.4	0.17	0.34	Human	0.26	22
Vasopressin	1084[c]	0.50	0.23	2.3	27.7	Human	5.54	18
LHRH	1182[c]	0.20	0.85	0.44	1.43	IPPSF	0.71	29
	1182[c]	2.00	2.12	1.62	2.13	Human	0.11	30
	1182[c]	3.00	2.12	11.4	15.0	Human	0.50	30
	1182[c]	4.00	2.12	24.5	32.1	Human	0.80	30

Compound								
[DTrp6-Pro9-NHEt] LHRH	1182c	0.50	2.12	0.23	0.30	Human	0.06	30
	1254c	0.10	0.06	0.86	39.8	HMS	39.8	27
	1254c	0.10	0.6	2.5	11.6	HMS	11.6	27
	1254c	0.10	3.0	5.0	4.63	HMS	4.63	27
	1254c	0.30	0.06	1.60	74.1	HMS	24.7	27
	1254c	0.30	0.6	5.8	26.9	HMS	8.95	27
	1254c	0.30	3.0	11.1	10.3	HMS	3.43	27
	1254c	0.50	0.06	2.2	102	HMS	20.4	27
	1254c	0.50	0.6	8.3	38.4	HMS	7.69	27
	1254c	0.50	3.0	13.6	12.6	HMS	2.52	27
	1254c	0.50	24.0	19.3	2.23	HMS	0.45	27
Nafarelin	1321c	0.16	0.76	0.14	0.52	HMS	0.33	34
	1321c	0.31	0.76	0.44	1.62	HMS	0.52	34
	1321c	0.47	0.76	0.53	1.95	HMS	0.42	34
	1321c	0.63	0.76	1.01	3.70	HMS	0.59	34
	1321c	0.63	0.38	0.25	1.83	HMS	0.29	34
	1321c	0.63	1.51	0.34	0.63	HMS	0.10	34
	1321c	0.63	2.27	0.21	0.25	HMS	0.04	34
	1321c	0.31	0.07	1.14	42.1	Human	13.7	35
	1321c	0.31	0.38	0.79	5.78	Human	1.83	35
	1321c	0.31	0.76	0.25	0.91	Human	0.29	35
	1321c	0.63	0.07	1.88	69.1	Human	10.9	35
	1321c	0.63	0.38	1.17	8.57	Human	1.36	35
	1321c	0.63	0.76	0.43	1.59	Human	0.25	35
Carboxy inulin	5200b	0.32	0.17	2.3d	2.00	HMS	0.62	1
	5200b	3.20	0.17	6.0d	0.52	HMS	0.02	1

a Zwitterion or neutral molecule.
b Anion.
c Cation.
d Calculated from the volume flux across the skin (μL/cm² h).

e Background electrolyte = NaCl.
f Background electrolyte = CaCl2.
g HMS = hairless mouse skin; NuRat = nude rat; NuMS = nude mice.

It is immediately obvious that, not only is there variability for any one compound as measured by different investigators, or by the same investigators at different times (no doubt due, at least in part, to the different experimental conditions employed), but that there is also no obvious relationship between molecular size and normalized flux. In addition to the confounding effects of the inconsistent experimental conditions used, of course, there is the issue of mechanism, i.e., electrorepulsion vs. electro-osmosis. In the former case, an inverse relationship between ionic mobility and size is predicted; in the latter, one anticipates that transport should be essentially independent of size, at least up to the point at which the molecular dimensions approach those of the most-constricted point of the pathway followed. As the dominant mechanism of transport almost certainly changes with size, it follows that the unraveling of a clear dependence of peptide flux upon molecular size is an extremely challenging objective; at the very least, it is essential that the fluxes of a series of peptides of increasing size, but fixed charge (and without significant skin association), be measured under identical conditions. At this time, no such systematic (yet fundamental) study has been undertaken. The closest approach to this type of investigation has involved determination of the normalized iontophoretic fluxes of a range of negatively charged compounds across hairless mouse skin *in vitro*; the anionic compounds were two amino acids, several acetylated amino acids, three tripeptides, AMP, ATP, GTP, and imido-GTP, and some negatively charged monomeric insulin analogs.[3,4,44,45,74] All experiments were conducted under very similar conditions at pH 7.4, and approximately the same constant current density. A normalized flux for chloride ion was also determined from another laboratory[81] and compared with these other data. Figure 7.7 plots the normalized fluxes as a function of molecular weight and shows that, as predicted for purely electrorepulsive iontophoresis, there is a general downward trend in transport with increasing molecular size (all other factors being maintained constant).

Likewise, with respect to purely electro-osmotic iontophoresis, the relationship between the normalized anodic iontophoretic fluxes of neutral compounds and their lipophilicity (as measured by the octanol–water partition coefficient, P) has been reported.[3,4,63] Under essentially consistent experimental conditions, it was found that electrotransport was *independent* of lipophilicity over five orders of magnitude of P, and it was concluded, therefore, that the environment of the iontophoretic transport pathway must be predominately aqueous in nature.

The charge on a molecule is clearly an important determinant of its iontophoretic flux rate. The sign of the charge will specify whether the transport mechanism is purely electrorepulsion (for anions) or a combination of electrorepulsion and electro-osmosis (for cations). That is, because of the skin permselectivity, a cation will transport better than a comparably sized anion, as has been shown for amino acids and tripeptides.[3,4,63] However, with respect to positively charged peptides (and indeed the other species as well) the situation is not quite so simple for at least two reasons. (1) To increase the number of positive charges on a peptide may necessitate the pH to be changed (i.e., decreased); this in theory, may diminish electro-osmosis, as the negativity of the skin is being neutralized by increasing $[H^+]$, and hence the overall electrotransport may be in fact be reduced. (2) An increased positive charge on a peptide may cause it to become more tightly associated with the membrane, and

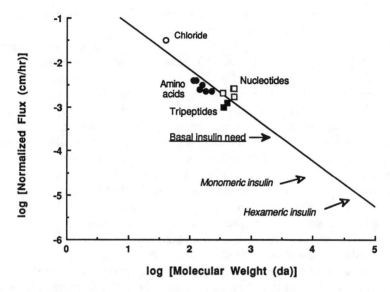

FIGURE 7.7 Normalized flux (iontophoretic flux in nmol/h/cm^2 divided by donor concentration of permeant in nmol/cm^3) as a function of molecular weight for the cathodal delivery of several anionic species across hairless mouse skin *in vitro* (current density $\approx$ 0.4 mA/cm^2; background electrolyte 25 mM HEPES buffer (133 mM NaCl); pH 7.4. The approximate values of normalized flux of monomeric and hexameric insulin are shown together with the value which is needed to satisfy the basal need of the drug in a patient with diabetes. (Results are redrawn from References 3, 4, 44, 74, and 81.)

thus produce a more substantial reservoir and decrease the rate at which steady-state flux might be achieved. As has already been discussed above, there are examples in the literature[6] of peptides which are iontophoresed more efficiently as neutral species at high pH ($\approx$8) than as cations under more acidic conditions ($\approx$pH 4).

Finally, it should be noted that isolectric focusing and capillary zone electrophoresis have been suggested as model systems with which relative peptide iontophoretic flux might be predicted. Certainly, these techniques can permit the effects of many important variables (e.g., pH, ionic strength, etc.) to be examined simply and rapidly, without the use of complicated *in vitro* and/or *in vivo* experimental setups.[71] While application of this idea to LHRH transport has been described,[75] there remains no validation of the overall utility of the approach in any practical or fundamental sense.

7.3.2 EXPERIMENTAL CONDITIONS: pH AND BACKGROUND ELECTROLYTE

The pH of the donor solution or electrode formulation can affect the electrotransport of a peptide in at least three different ways: (1) the pH can determine the ionization state of the peptide, depending upon the overall pI and the respective pK_a values of the charged amino acid residues in the structure; (2) as discussed above, the permselectivity of the skin is pH dependent; and (3) because of the high mobilities of H$^+$

and OH⁻ ions, their competition as charged carriers increases dramatically as the pH moves away from neutrality.

The net charge on the skin depends upon the pH of the electrolyte solutions on either side of the membrane. *In vitro*, skin permselectivity can be reversed by using donor and receptor solutions at pH 4;[66] in such circumstances, electro-osmotic flow is from cathode to anode. These conditions, while superficially attractive for negative peptides, cannot, however, be realized *in vivo* where the "receptor" phase is always at pH 7.4. Even with the asymmetric arrangement (pH 4 donor, pH 7.4 receptor) *in vitro*, convective flow overall remains anode to cathode.[66] It should be noted that iontophoresis of AVP (pI = 10.8) into rats *in vivo* produced an antidiuretic response when donor solutions spanning a wide range of pH (4 to 8) were used.[20-21] On the other hand, iontophoresis of salmon calcitonin[24] (pI = 6.5) resulted in a significant effect on plasma calcium concentration only when a donor solution at pH 4 was subjected to iontophoresis; no effects were observed at higher pHs (5.5, 7, and 8).

Given that all ions present in an iontophoresis system compete to carry the charge across the membrane, it follows that decreasing the ionic strength of the electrolyte composition of the electrode formulation (all other factors being constant) should lead to increased drug flux. In addition, increased electro-osmotic delivery (of course, from the anode) is also anticipated due to increased volume flow at low ionic strength.[1,62,65] There have been several studies of the effect of ionic strength on peptide iontophoresis,[11,15,21,22,32,40] and, in general, the results confirm that higher electrotransport occurs at lower concentration of electrolyte. The idea has been exploited, for example, by using polymeric buffers[8] to increase the iontophoresis of dTLP (desamino-tyrosil-lysyl-prolineamide) and TRH. While the preceding arguments are true for constant current iontophoresis, opposite behavior (for different reasons) can be observed when using a constant voltage protocol. For example, with the analog of GRF Ro 23-7861,[13] it was shown that increasing the buffer concentration (or, indeed, the strength of background electrolyte, or the current density) resulted in more ions in the skin, thereby lowering the membrane resistance which, in turn, provoked a higher current density (and, hence, delivery).

Returning to the constant current situation, and the use of Ag/AgCl electrodes, attention is drawn to *in vitro* diffusion studies in which the receptor solution is continuously perfused with an electrolyte solution at physiological pH (i.e., comparable to *in vivo* conditions). Due to the skin permselectivity, and the presence of only finite amounts of Na⁺ and Cl⁻ in the donor electrode chambers at $t = 0$, the concentration of NaCl in the anode falls with the time of current passage, while that in the cathode increases. It follows that delivery of a cation should increase with time, while that of an anion will fall. Data with simple, singly charged positive and negative amino acids are in agreement with this analysis.[3]

Most published studies of peptide iontophoresis have used either Ag/AgCl or Pt electrodes. The former are preferred as they avoid problems associated with pH changes caused by the electrolysis of water at Pt electrodes. Changes in pH, in addition to the effects identified at the beginning of this section, can also result in peptide degradation and exaggerated local skin irritation. The limitations of Ag/AgCl electrodes are (1) the requirement of a finite Cl⁻ concentration at the anode to more than satisfy the electrochemical reaction for the duration of current passage[76]; (2) the possibility of electrochemical reaction of the peptide at the Ag/AgCl surface; and (3) the incompatibility of the peptide (e.g., poor stability) in solutions containing, for example, high concentrations of salt. The two latter problems have sometimes been resolved by isolating the peptide from the electrode by means of either a salt bridge[27,33,34,61] or an ion-selective membrane[25] (e.g., salmon calcitonin and LHRH). However, significant leakage of ions from a salt bridge can occur and alter thereby the observed electrotransport.[33] The difficulties with Pt (and other, for example, stainless steel[14]) electrodes have been well documented, and large pH changes during iontophoresis have been reported on numerous occasions.[10,13,19,32] To reduce this problem, either the pH of the electrode solutions must be frequently or continuously adjusted[6] or very strong buffers (which introduce competitive ions) must be used.[16,32] Even so, degradation of buserelin,[32] CCK-8 analog,[36] LHRH,[31] salmon calcitonin,[26] and AVP[15] during iontophoresis from Pt electrodes has been reported. In addition to the effects of pH changes, electrochemical reactions and enzymatic degradation have been implicated.

Finally, with respect to the practical realization of a useful iontophoretic device, it is noted that almost all the work reported to date has involved aqueous electrode formulations. While these are clearly appropriate for fundamental research, a more convenient vehicle (e.g., a gel) will be necessary for a clinically useful device. The literature, however, reveals only limited information concerning peptide iontophoresis from such delivery systems.[5,17,19,31,32]

7.4 IN VIVO RESULTS

The majority of *in vivo* work performed has involved various animals models. At this time, there have been no systematic studies of peptide iontophoresis *in vivo*. There are a number of reports concerning insulin, and this subject has been very recently reviewed in depth.[77] The efficacy of insulin iontophoresis has most often been evaluated from the lowering of blood glucose levels in small rodents.[51-54] For example, in rats (haired and hairless), anodal iontophoresis of the peptide at pH 3.68 resulted in better glucose lowering than cathodal delivery at higher pH (5.3, 7.1, and 8). The authors of this work suggested that the increased delivery at lower pH was the result of diminished peptide self-association that occurs under more basic conditions. However, given the discussion above concerning electrorepulsion vs. electro-osmotic mechanisms of electrotransport, it is possible that the electro-osmotic delivery of insulin from the anode at low pH is more efficient than its electrorepulsive input (against the convective flow) from the cathode at higher pH. The form of the current profile (e.g., direct vs. pulsed current at different frequencies) has also been examined and some differences observed. However, such behavior has not been observed by other investigators using different solutes,[78] and further confirmation with insulin is therefore necessary before these former data can be attributed significant weight. Successful lowering of hyperglycemia in rabbits[50] has also been achieved iontophoretically, but only after the stratum corneum had been physically damaged! Furthermore, as inert electrodes were used, the cathodal (delivery) solution pH increased from 7 to 12 in a 3-h period! Similar results reported elsewhere (i.e., a hypoglycemic effect and a large pH shift due to water hydrolysis), again in rabbits, have been achieved without prior disruption of the stratum corneum.[48] It is important to remember in these studies that lowering of blood sugar in small animals requires delivery of a relatively small amount of insulin. If the deliveries achieved are transferred to humans, then the predicted input is 10 to 100 times below that necessary to provide even a basal level of the hormone.[44,45] Only one report of insulin iontophoresis in humans has appeared[49]; however, as the work was targeted toward the treatment of cystic fibrosis, no information concerning systemic insulin levels was given.

The *ad hoc* nature of much of the other *in vivo* experiments can be illustrated by the following examples:

(1) An excellent *in vitro* to *in vivo* correlation for iontophoresis of the tripeptide Thr-Lys-Pro has been obtained.[5] The *in vitro* flux was shown to be completely consistent with the apparent urinary excretion rate of the peptide following *in vivo* delivery to hairless rats. Pretreatment of rats with an iontophoretic current followed by passive application of the peptide also resulted in enhanced delivery. While current passage *in vivo* caused some reddening of the electrode sites, no histological changes were detected.

(2) Iontophoresis of GRF (1-44) (MW 5040) into hairless guinea pigs[14] resulted in steady-state plasma levels of ≈ 0.2 ng/mL, corresponding to an estimated input rate of ≈ 3.16 µg/h.

(3) Octreotide, a somatostatin analog, was iontophoresed into rabbits *in vivo* and resulted in plasma levels that were proportional to the applied current delivery.[12] Plasma levels declined quickly upon current termination. However, as noted before, the area under the plasma concentration vs. time curve was not proportional to the peptide concentration administered (see Figure 7.5). Notably, reasonable delivery rates were achieved with modest current densities (50 to 150 µA/cm^2).

(4) Two studies have measured calcitonin iontophoresis *in vivo*. Human calcitonin delivery (with both pulsed and direct current) to hairless rats[26] lowered serum calcium, but the effects were not linear with respect to either current density or time of current application. In "hairy" rats, iontophoresis of salmon calcitonin again elicited the desired pharmacological effect.[24] This investigation also examined how delivery of the intact peptide was influenced by pH and the presence of several protease inhibitors.

Finally, there is an increasing body of knowledge concerning *in vivo* iontophoresis of LHRH and its analog, leuprolide. The IPPSF technique has been used successfully as a tool with which to predict LHRH plasma concentrations during iontophoresis of the peptide *in vivo* in pigs.[28] In the latter experiments, not only did iontophoresis lead to elevated LHRH concentrations in the blood, there were also concomitant increases in LH and FSH (follicle-stimulating hormone) levels, showing that the delivered peptide was an active species. Plasma levels of the peptide fell rapidly once iontophoresis was terminated. Experiments with the IPPSF have also shown[29] that LHRH can form a significant depot in the skin, with 1.4% of the dose being found in the tissue (SC + underlying skin + subcutaneous tissue) 2 h after termination of current flow. During the initial iontophoresis period, it should be noted, only 0.7% of the dose was delivered across the IPPSF into the perfusate. When this initial treatment protocol was followed by a second iontophoretic episode, significantly more LHRH was delivered "systemically" than could be explained by the accumulation during the first dosing interlude (a second iontophoretic episode only mobilized 2% of the depot). The exact reason for the finding remains unknown at this time; alteration in skin permeability properties or peptide binding are possible contributory factors. The important message, though, is that peptide iontophoretic devices, which are intended to provide intermittent periods of drug delivery, quite possibly through the same skin site, will need to be examined and validated very carefully for nonlinearity (or rather its absence) with respect to drug input. Local "side effects" should also be examined; for example, in the IPPSF study, some histological changes were seen in 15% of the active electrodes considered.

The LHRH analog leuprolide has been iontophoresed into human volunteers,[38,39] provoking an increase in LH levels. Despite the fact that considerable variability was observed, these results are nevertheless remarkable for the fact that the pharmacodynamic changes were elicited by passage of a maximum of 0.2 mA over 70 cm^2 (approximately 3.1 µA/cm^2), using electrode "patches" containing 1 mL of Leupron® ([leuprolide] = 5 mg/mL). Passive transdermal delivery was inefficient; iontophoresis matched subcutaneous injection. The local effects of the iontophoresis were very mild: slight erytheme at the electrode sites that resolved quickly after current termination in 6 of 13 subjects, and a small tingling sensation during current passage in 2 of 13 volunteers.

Another human study[40] with leuprolide examined the effects of drug concentration and ionic strength on iontophoretic delivery (see Figure 7.4). The highest efficiency was observed at the lowest leuprolide concentration and lowest ionic strength. The effect of changes in the donor solution composition on leuprolide plasma concentration was greater than that on LH and testosterone levels, presumably reflecting the importance of interindividual differences in pharmacological response. It further shows that pharmacological measurements are insufficient end points with which to estimate iontophoretic fluxes and they can "blur" the effects of formulation changes on the absolute quantity of peptide delivery.

7.5 METABOLISM

A major problem with respect to the nonparenteral delivery of peptides is presystemic metabolism. For example, the oral bioavailability of peptides is very poor due to their degradation in the GI tract prior to absorption. Of course, this problem explains, in large part, why other administration routes are under consideration, but begs the further question of metabolism at other locations in the organism. To address this issue, for example, leucine aminopeptidase activities in homogenates from rectal, dermal, buccal, intestinal, and nasal tissues of the rat were compared.[79] The results showed that the dermal homogenate had the lowest aminopeptidase activity, although normalization of the data by tissue protein content indicated that the skin was equivalent to rectal and nasal tissues, higher than the buccal mucosa but lower than the intestine. Overall, these data suggested that the transdermal route could be a feasible route for peptide administration if the penetration rate were sufficiently fast.

In an extensive work with leu-enkephalin,[80] the activities of aminopeptidases, endopeptidases, and carboxipeptidases in hairless mouse skin were examined. At pH 7, all peptide bonds were cleaved during passive permeation of leu-enkephalin. Blocking the terminal amino group, however, protected the peptide against endopeptidase activity. Notably, it was shown that the receptor phase had significant enzyme activity only 5 min after incubation with the skin, suggesting that leakage of enzymes from the tissue had occurred. Furthermore, the proteolytic activity of a skin homogenate was different from that of freshly excised skin, and the actions of peptidase inhibitors in these two circumstances were not equivalent. These findings show some of the problems associated with the performance of meaningful metabolism experiments *in vitro*. First, during the transport process, does the peptide encounter different enzymes (or levels of enzymes) *in vitro* than it does *in vivo* due, for example, to artifactual release of enzymes during the tissue preparation process? Second, how can the *in vitro* results be confirmed *in vivo*? Third, are the data from rat, for instance, relevant to those that would be found in humans? How does one ensure human skin viability *in vitro* for a sufficient period to ensure "meaningful data"? Without question, more information concerning metabolic activity in iontophoretic pathways is required. However, the techniques necessary to provide these data unambiguously are not yet at hand.

Nevertheless, metabolism of peptides during iontophoresis *in vitro* also occurs. For small peptides, metabolism has been found to be quite modest.[3-6] For larger species, however, more significant metabolism has been seen. For example, 60% of vasopressin delivered by iontophoresis through human skin *in vitro* was metabolized;[18] contact simply with the receptor solution that had bathed with the underside of the skin was sufficient to cause peptide breakdown; i.e., even if vasopressin crossed the skin unscathed, it could still be broken down before its transport was recorded.

For LHRH,[31] an important metabolism was found at pH 5 and pH 7 but not at pH 3 during iontophoresis through hairless rat skin *in vitro*. LHRH was found to be completely metabolized in hairless mouse skin[27] at pH 7.0. Nevertheless, it should be noted that, despite the important metabolism of LHRH reported *in vitro*, iontophoresis of the peptide *in vivo* in pigs caused LH and FSH levels to increase showing that intact LHRH[28] was delivered. The LHRH analog [D-Trp[6],Pro[9]-NHEt]LHRH, on the other hand, was more resistant to enzymatic degradation[27] while metabolism of nafarelin at pH 7 was also significant.[33]

An interesting strategy to circumvent the metabolism problem is to deliver simultaneously by iontophoresis both the peptide and an enzyme inhibitor.[20,24] Salmon calcitonin[24] and vasopressin[20] were iontophoresed *in vivo* to rats in the presence and absence of three different protease inhibitors: camostat mesilate, soybean trypsin inhibitor, and aprotinin. The pharmacological effects, changes in calcium plasma levels, and antidiuretic response, respectively, were measured. Aprotinin and camostat mesilate enhanced the hypocalcemic effect observed, while soybean trypsin inhibitor did not. For vasopressin, only camostat mesilate was effective as an inhibitor and enhanced the antidiuretic effect. Apart from their differences in antiprotease activity, other characteristics of the inhibitors may explain the differences in the observed results: Camostat mesylate (MW 495) and aprotinin (MW 6500) are cations, while soybean trypsine inhibitor is a high-molecular-weight (8000) anion.

7.6 SUMMARY

It can be concluded, without question, that iontophoresis can succesfully promote peptide transport across the skin. However, the diversity of the molecules studied, and the enormous range of experimental conditions used, render more-detailed deductions much more difficult to draw. Clearly, there is a need for the development of more comprehensive structure–penetration relationships, and the differentiation of electrorepulsive and electro-osmotic mechanisms of transport has important implications for the eventual development of practical peptide iontophoretic systems.

The peptidase metabolic activity of the skin must be characterized, as, more generally, must the chronic effects of current passage on the skin itself. Nevertheless, it is reasonable to suggest that the knowledge that has been accumulated to date supports the feasibility and practicality of iontophoresis for potent peptides of appropiate pharmacodynamic profile. Optimization of the enhancement strategy will require significant further research and the creative transfer of this science to technology development.

ACKNOWLEDGMENTS

We thank our past and present colleagues for their continued advice and discussion; in particular, the input of Dr. Philip Green made this chapter much easier to prepare. Our work in this area has been supported by the U.S. National Institutes of Health and by Becton Dickinson.

REFERENCES

1. Pikal, M. J. and Shah, S., Transport mechanisms in iontophoresis. III. An experimental study of the contributions of electroosmotic flow and permeability change in transport of low and high molecular weight solutes, *Pharm. Res.,* 7, 222, 1990.
2. Wearley, L. L., Tojo, K., and Chien, Y, W., A numerical approach to study the effect of binding on the iontophoretic transport of a series of amino acids, *J. Pharm. Sci.,* 79, 992, 1990.
3. Green, P. G., Hinz, R. S., Cullander, C., Yamane, G., and Guy, R. H., Iontophoretic delivery of amino acids and amino acid derivatives across the skin "in vitro," *Pharm. Res.,* 8, 1113, 1991.
4. Green, P. G., Hinz, R. S., Kim, A., Szoka, F. C., and Guy, R. H., Iontophoretic delivery of a series of tripeptides across the skin in vitro, *Pharm. Res.,* 8, 1121, 1991.
5. Green, P. G., Shroot, B., Bernerd, F., Pilgrim, W. R., and Guy, R. H., In vitro and in vivo iontophoresis of a tripeptide across nude rat skin, *J. Controlled Release,* 20, 209, 1992.
6. Burnette, R. R. and Marrero, D., Comparison between the iontophoretic and passive transport of thyrotropin releasing hormone across excised nude mouse skin, *J. Pharm. Sci.,* 75, 738, 1992.
7. Jadoul, A., Hanchard, C., Thysman, S., and Préat, V., Quantification and localization of fentanyl and TRH delivered by iontophoresis in the skin, *Int. J. Pharm.,* 120, 221, 1995.
8. Sarpotdar, P. P. and Daniels, C. R., Use of polymeric buffers to facilitate iontophoretic transport of drugs, *Pharm. Res.,* 7 (Suppl.), S-185, 1990.

9. Sarpotdar, P. P., Daniels, C. R., Liversidge, G. G., and Sternson, L. A., Facilitated iontophoretic delivery of thyrotropin releasing hormone (TRH) across cadaver skin by optimization of formulation variables, *Pharm. Res.,* 6 (Suppl.), S-107, 1989.

10. Gupta, S. K., Kumar, S., Bolton, S., Behl C. R., and Malick, A. W., Optimization of iontophoretic transdermal delivery of a peptide and a non-peptide drug, *J. Controlled Release,* 30, 253, 1994.

11. Clemessy, M., Couarraze, G., Bevan, B., and Puisieux, F., Mechanisms involved in iontophoretic transport of angiotensin, *Pharm. Res.,* 12, 998, 1995.

12. Lau, D. T. W., Sharkey, J. W., Petryk, L., Mancuso, F. A., Yu, Z., and Tse, F. L. S., Effect of current magnitude and drug concentration on iontophoretic delivery of octreotide acetate (Sandostatin®) in the rabbit, *Pharm. Res.,* 11, 1742, 1994.

13. Kumar, S., Char, H., Patel, S., Piemontese, D., Iqbal, K., Malick, A. W., Neugroschel, E., and Behl, C. R., Effect of iontophoresis on in vitro skin permeation of an analogue of growth hormone releasing hormone in the hairless guinea pig model, *J. Pharm. Sci.,* 81, 635, 1992.

14. Kumar, S., Char, H., Patel, S., Piemontese, D., Malick, A. W., Iqbal, K., Neugroschel, E., and Behl, C. R., In vivo transdermal iontophoretic delivery of growth hormone releasing factor GRF (1-44) in hairless guinea pigs, *J. Controlled Release,* 18, 213, 1992.

15. Lelawongs, P., Liu, J. C., Siddiqui, O., and Chien, Y. W., Transdermal iontophoretic delivery of arginine-vasopressin. (I): Physicochemical considerations, *Int. J. Pharm.,* 56, 13, 1989.

16. Lelawongs, P., Liu, J. C., and Chien, Y. W., Transdermal iontophoretic delivery of arginine-vasopressin. (II): Evaluation of electrical and operational factors, *Int. J. Pharm.,* 61, 179, 1989.

17. Banga, A. K. and Chien, Y. W., Hydrogel-based Iontotherapeutic delivery devices for transdermal delivery of peptide/protein drugs, *Pharm. Res.,* 10, 697, 1993.

18. Banga, A. K., Katakam, M., and Mitra, R., Transdermal iontophoretic delivery and degradation of vasopressin across human cadaver skin, *Int. J. Pharm.,* 116, 211, 1995.

19. Brady, A. B., Corish, J., and Corrigan, O. I., Passive and electrically assisted transdermal delivery of desamino-8-D-arginine vasopressin in vitro from a gel matrix, in *Prediction of Percutaneous Penetration,* Scott, R. C., Guy, R. H., Hadgraft, J., and Boddé, H. E., Eds., Vol. 2, STS Publishing, Cardiff, U.K., 1991, 401.

20. Morimoto, K., Iwakura, Y., Miyazaki, M., and Nakatani, E., Effects of proteolytic enzyme inhibitors of enhancement of transdermal iontophoretic delivery of vasopressin and an analog in rats, *Int. J. Pharm.,* 81, 119, 1992.

21. Iwakura, Y. and Morimoto, K., Transdermal iontophoretic delivery of vasopressin and its analogue in rats, *S.T.P. Pharm. Sci.,* 1, 387, 1991.

22. Craane-van Hinsberg, W. H. M., Bax, L., Flinterman, N. H. M., Verhoef, J., Junginger, H. E., and Bodde, H. E., Iontophoresis of a model peptide across human skin in vitro: effects of iontophoresis protocol, pH and ionic strength on peptide flux and skin impedance, *Pharm. Res.,* 11, 1296, 1994.

23. Craane-van Hinsberg, W. H. M., Coos Verhoef, J., Box, L. J., Junginger, H. E., and Bodde, H. E., Role of appendages in skin resistance and iontophoretic peptide flux: human versus snake skin, *Pharm. Res.,* 12, 1506, 1995.

24. Morimoto, K., Iwakura, Y., Nakatani, E., Miyazaki, M., and Tojima, H., Effects of proteolytic enzyme inhibitors as absorption enhancers on the transdermal iontophoretic delivery of calcitonin in rats, *J. Pharm. Pharmacol.,* 44, 216, 1992.

25. Hager, D. F., Mancuso, F. A., Nazareno, J. P., Sharkey, J. W., and Siverly, J. R., Evaluation of a cultured skin equivalent as a model membrane for iontophoretic transport, *J. Controlled Release*, 30, 117, 1994.
26. Thysman, S., Hanchard, C., and Préat, V., Human calcitonin delivery in rats by iontophoresis, *J. Pharm. Pharmacol.*, 46, 725, 1994.
27. Miller, L. L., Kolaskie, C. J., Smith, G. A., and Riviere, J., Transdermal iontophoresis of gonadotropin releasing hormone (LHRH) and two analogues, *J. Pharm. Sci.*, 79, 490, 1990.
28. Heit, M. C., Williams, P. L., Jayes, F. L., Chang, S. K., and Riviere, J. E., Transdermal iontophoretic peptide delivery: in vitro and in vivo studies with luteinizing hormone releasing hormone, *J. Pharm. Sci.*, 83, 240, 1993.
29. Heit, M. C., Monteiro-Riviere, N. A., Jayes, F. L., and Riviere, J. E., Transdermal iontophoretic delivery of luteinizing hormone releasing hormone (LHRH): effect of repeated administration, *Pharm. Res.*, 11, 1000, 1994.
30. Bommannan, D. B., Tamada, J., Leung, L., and Potts, R. O., Effect of electroporation on transdermal iontophoretic delivery of luteinizing hormone releasing hormone (LHRH) in vitro, *Pharm. Res.*, 11, 1809, 1994.
31. Chen, L. H. and Chien, Y. W., Development of a skin permeation cell to simulate clinical study of iontophoretic transdermal delivery, *Drug Dev. Ind. Pharm.*, 20, 935, 1994.
32. Knoblauch, P. and Moll, F., In vitro pulsatile and continuous transdermal delivery of buserelin by iontophoresis, *J. Controlled Release*, 26, 203, 1993.
33. Delgado-Charro, M. B. and Guy, R. H., Iontophoretic delivery of nafarelin across the skin, *Int. J. Pharm.*, 117, 165, 1995.
34. Delgado-Charro, M. B., Rodriguez-Bayón, A. M., and Guy, R. H., Iontophoresis of nafarelin: effects of current density and concentration on electrotransport in vitro, *J. Controlled Release*, 35, 35, 1995.
35. Rodriguez-Bayón, A. M. and Guy, R. H., Iontophoresis of nafarelin across human skin in vitro, *Pharm. Res.*, 13, 798, 1996.
36. Srinivasan, V., Su, M., Higuchi, W. I., and Behl, C. R., Iontophoresis of polypeptides: effect of ethanol pretreatment of human skin, *J. Pharm. Sci.*, 79, 588, 1990.
37. Hoogstraate, A. J., Srinivasan, V., Sims, S. M., and Higuchi, W. I., Iontophoretic enhancement of peptides: behaviour of leuprolide versus model permeants, *J. Controlled Release*, 31, 41, 1994.
38. Meyer, B. R., Kreis, W., Eschbah, J., O'Mara, V., Rosen, S., and Sibalis, D., Successful transdermal administration of therapeutic doses of a polypeptide to normal volunteeers, *Clin. Pharmacol. Ther.*, 44, 607, 1988.
39. Meyer, B. R., Kreis, W., Eschbach, J., O'Mara, V., Rosen, S., and Sibalis, D., Transdermal versus subcutaneous leuprolide: A comparison of acute pharmacodynamic effect, *Clin. Pharmacol. Ther.*, 48, 340, 1990.
40. Fu Lu, M., Lee, D., Carlson, R., Rao, G. S., Hui, H. W., Adjei, L., Herrin, M., Sundberg, D., and Hsu, L., The effects of formulation variables on iontophoretic transdermal delivery of leuprolide to humans, *Drug Dev. Ind. Pharm.*, 19, 1557, 1993.
41. Burton, S. A. and Ferber, R. H., Effect of current density, AC frequency, and pH on electrically enhanced transdermal sucrose and methionine enkephalin (MENK) flux, *Pharm. Res.*, 6(Suppl.), S-107, 1989.
42. Banga, A. K. and Chien, Y. W. Characterization of in vitro transdermal iontophoretic delivery of insulin, *Drug Dev. Ind. Pharm.*, 19, 2069, 1993.

43. Srinivasan, V., Higuchi, W. I., Sims, S, M., Ghanem, A. H., and Behl, C. R., Transdermal iontophoretic drug delivery: mechanistic analysis and application to polypeptide delivery, *J. Pharm. Sci.,* 78, 370, 1989.

44. Langkjær, L., Brange, J., Grodsky, G. M., and Guy, R. H., Transdermal delivery of monomeric insulin analogues by iontophoresis. *Proc. Int. Symp. Control. Rel. Biact. Mater.,* 21, 172, 1994.

45. Langkjær, L., Brange, J., Grodsky, G. M., and Guy, R. H., Transdermal delivery of monomeric insulin analogues by iontophoresis, paper presented at 29th Annual Meeting of the European Association for the Study of Diabetes, Istanbul, September 6–9, 1993.

46. Thysman, S. and Preat, V., Influence of electrochemical factors on iontophoresis, in *Prediction of Percutaneous Penetration,* Scott, R. C., Guy, R. H., Hadgraft, J., and Bodde, H. E., Eds., Vol. 2, STS Publishing, Cardiff, U.K., 1991, 156.

47. Stephen, R. L., Petelenz, T. J., and Jacobsen, S. C., Potential novel methods for insulin administration: I. Iontophoresis, *Biomed. Biochim. Acta,* 43, 553, 1984.

48. Meyer, B. R., Katzeff, H. L., Eschbach, J. C., Trimmer, J., Zacharias, S. B., Rosen, S., and Sibalis, D., Transdermal delivery of human insulin to albino rabbits using electrical current, *Am. J. Med. Sci.,* 297, 321, 1989.

49. Shapiro, B. L., Pence, T. V., and Warwick, W. J., Insulin iontophoresis in cystic fibrosis, *Proc. Soc. Exp. Biol. Med.,* 149, 592, 1975.

50. Kari, B., Control of blood glucose levels in alloxan-diabetic rabbits by iontophoresis of insulin, *Diabetes,* 35, 217, 1986.

51. Liu, J. C., Sun, Y., Siddiqui, O., Chien, Y. W., Shi, W., and Li, J., Blood glucose control in diabetic rats by transdermal iontophoretic delivery of insulin, *Int. J. Pharm.,* 44, 197, 1988.

52. Chien, Y. W., Lelawongs, P., Siddiqui, O., Sun, Y., and Shi, W. M., Facilitated transdermal delivery of therapeutic peptides and proteins by iontophoretic delivery devices, *J. Controlled Release,* 13, 263, 1990.

53. Chien, Y. W., Siddiqui, O., Sun, Y., Shi, W. M., and Liu, J. C., Transdermal iontophoretic delivery of therapeutic peptides/proteins I: Insulin, *Ann. N.Y. Acad. Sci.,* 507, 32, 1987.

54. Siddiqui, O., Sun, Y., Liu, J., and Chien, Y. W., Facilitated transdermal transport of insulin, *J. Pharm. Sci.,* 76, 341, 1987.

55. Chien, Y. W., Siddiqui, O., Shi, W. M., Lelawongs, P., and Liu, J. C., Direct current iontophoretic transdermal delivery of peptide and protein drugs, *J. Pharm. Sci.,* 78, 376, 1989.

56. Hager, D. F., Mancuso, F. A., Nazareno, J. P., Sharkey, J. W., and Siverly, J. R., Evaluation of Testskin™ as a model membrane, *Proc. Int. Symp. Control. Rel. Mater.,* 19, 487, 1992.

57. Nestor, J. J., Ho, T. L., Tahilramani, R., McRae, G. I., and Vickery, B. H., Long acting LHRH agonists and antagonists, in *LHRH and Its Analogs,* Labrie, F., Belanger, A., and Dupont, A., Eds., Elsevier Science Publishers, Amsterdam, 1984, 24.

58. Oh, S. Y., Leung, L., Bommannan, D., Guy, R. H., and Potts, R. O., Effect of current, ionic strength and temperature on the electrical properties of skin, *J. Controlled Release,* 27, 115, 1993.

59. Kalia, Y. N. and Guy R. H., The electrical characteristics of human skin in vivo, *Pharm. Res.,* 12, 1605, 1995.

60. Ledger, P. W., Skin biological issues in electrically enhanced transdermal delivery, *Adv. Drug Delivery Rev.,* 9, 289, 1992.

61. Delgado-Charro, M. B. and Guy, R. H., Characterization of convective solvent flow during iontophoresis, *Pharm. Res.,* 11, 929, 1994.

62. Pikal, M. J., The role of electroosmotic flow in transdermal iontophoresis, *Adv. Drug Delivery Rev.*, 9, 201, 1992.
63. Green, P. G., Hinz, R. S., Kim, A., Cullander, C., Yamane, G., Szoka, F. C., and Guy, R. H., Transdermal iontophoresis of amino acids and peptides in vitro, *J. Controlled Release*, 21, 187, 1992.
64. Santi, P. and Guy, R. H., Reverse iontophoresis — parameters determining electroosmotic flow. II. Electrode chamber formulation, *J. Controlled Release*, 42, 29, 1996.
65. Santi, P. and Guy, R. H., Reverse iontophoresis — parameters determining electroosmotic flow. I. pH and ionic strength, *J. Controlled Release*, 38, 159, 1996.
66. Kim, A., Green, P. G., Rao, G., and Guy, R. H., Convective solvent flow across the skin during iontophoresis, *Pharm. Res.*, 10, 1315, 1993.
67. Rabel, S. R. and Stobaugh, J. F., Applications of capillary electrophoresis in pharmaceutical analyisis, *Pharm. Res.*, 10, 171, 1993.
68. Hirvonen, J. and Guy, R. H., Transdermal iontophoresis: modulation of electroosmosis by polypeptides, *J. Controlled Release*, 50, 283, 1998.
69. Hirvonen, J., Kalia, Y. N., and Guy, R. H., Transdermal delivery of peptides by iontophoresis, *Nature Biotech.*, 14, 1710, 1996.
70. Hirvonen, J. and Guy, R. H., Iontophoretic delivery across the skin: electroosmosis and its modulation by drug substances, *Pharm. Res.*, 14, 1258, 1997
71. VanOrman Huff, B., Liversidge, G. G., and McIntire, G. L., The electrophoretic mobility of tripeptides as a function of pH and ionic strength: comparison with iontophoretic flux data, *Pharm. Res.*, 12, 751, 1995.
72. Powell, M. F., Sanders, L. M., Rogerson, A., and Si, V., Parenteral peptide formulations: chemical and physical properties of native luteinizing hormone releasing hormone (LHRH) and hydrophobic analogues in aqueous solution, *Pharm. Res.*, 8, 1258, 1991.
73. Brand, R. M., Singh, P., Aspe-Carranza, E., Maibach, H. I., and Guy, R. H., Acute effects of iontophoresis on human skin in vivo: cutaneous blood flow and transepidermal water loss measurements, *Eur. J. Pharm. Biopharm.*, 43, 133, 1997.
74. Van der Geest, R., Hueber, F., Szoka, F. C. Jr, and Guy, R. H., Iontophoresis of bases, nucleosides and nucleotides, *Pharm. Res.*, 13, 551, 1996.
75. Heit, M. C., McFarland, A., Bock, R., and Riviere, J. E., Isoelectric focusing and capillary zone eletrophoretic studies using luteinizing hormone releasing hormone and its analog, *J. Pharm. Sci.*, 85, 654, 1994.
76. Cullander, C., Rao, G., and Guy, R. H., Why silver/silver chloride? Criteria for iontophoresis electrodes, in *Prediction of Percutaneous Penetration*, Brain, K. R., James, V. J., and Walters, K. A., Eds., Vol. 3b, STS Publishing, Cardiff, U.K., 1993, 381.
77. Sage, B. H., Insulin iontophoresis, in *Protein Delivery — Physical Systems*, Sanders, L. M. and Hendron, R. W., Eds., Plenum Press, New York, 1997, 319.
78. Hirvonen, J., Hueber, F., and Guy R. H., Current profile regulates iontophoretic delivery of amino acids across the skin, *J. Controlled Release*, 37, 239, 1995.
79. Zhou, X. H. and Li Wan Po, A., Comparison of enzymic activities of tissues lining portals of drugs absorption using the rat as a model, *Int. J. Pharm.*, 62, 259, 1990.
80. Choi, H., Flynn, G. L., and Amidon, G. L., Transdermal delivery of bioactive peptides: the effect of n-decylmethyl sulfoxide, pH and inhibitors on enkephalin metabolism and transport., *Pharm. Res.*, 7, 1099, 1990.
81. Burnette, R. R. and Ongpipattanakul, B., Characterization of the permselective properties of excised human skin during iontophoresis, *J. Pharm. Sci.*, 76, 765, 1987.

Section III
Technical Applications

8 Glucose Monitoring Using Electroosmotic Transdermal Extraction

Janet A. Tamada and Russell O. Potts

CONTENTS

8.1 INTRODUCTION

Results from the Diabetes Care and Complications Trial show that tight glucose control significantly reduces the long-term complications of diabetes mellitus.[1] In that study, frequent self-testing of glucose and insulin administration resulted in a significant reduction in long-term complications. That protocol, however, also resulted in a threefold increase in the frequency of hypoglycemic incidents. Currently, self-testing requires a drop of blood for each measurement. The pain and inconvenience of self-testing, along with the fear and danger of hypoglycemia has led to poor patient acceptance of a tight control regimen, despite the clear long-term advantages. A continuously worn, noninvasive method to measure glucose periodically would provide a convenient and comfortable means of frequent self-testing.[2,3] Such a device could also alert the user of low serum glucose levels, thereby reducing the incidence of hypoglycemia.[4,5]

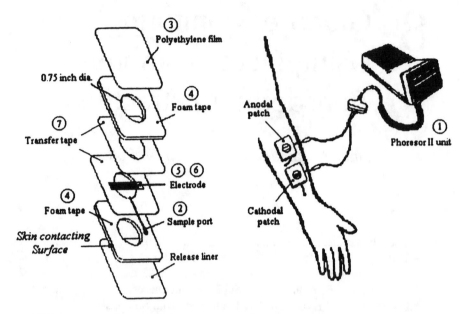

FIGURE 8.1   Schematic of extraction reservoir and electroosmotic extraction setup.

Guy et al.[6-8] demonstrated a method to transport glucose through the skin using low-level electrical current. Traditionally, application of low-level current has been used to deliver charged molecules into the body.[9,10] However, transport occurs in both directions; hence, substances transported from beneath the skin can be extracted into a collection reservoir for analysis. To provide a quantitative measurement, the flux of glucose extracted across the skin must correlate with serum glucose in a predictive manner. The results presented here show a quantitative relationship between serum and transdermally extracted glucose in human subjects.[11,12]

8.2   METHODS

8.2.1   Electroosmotic Extraction and Analysis

Two adhesive collection patches, each containing an aqueous collection chamber with an Ag/AgCl electrode, were applied to the volar surface of the forearm of the subject (Figure 8.1). The collection chambers had an extraction surface area of 2.85 cm² and a volume of 0.4 mL per patch. The extraction solution was either unbuffered 0.45% sodium chloride in water, U.S.P. (Baxter), or a 1:9 (v:v) mixture of 0.45% sodium chloride with 5% sodium bicarbonate, U.S.P. (Baxter), at pH between 8.2 and 8.8. The extraction solution was introduced into the chambers with a 1-mL syringe.

Glucose collection was achieved using either a direct current (DC) protocol or an alternating polarity (AP) protocol with a half-cycle duration of either 15 or 7.5 min. For all protocols, 0.32 mA/cm² (0.9 mA) was applied for 15 min, followed by a 5-min rest interval, during which the solution in the collection reservoir was removed, placed into tared vials and weighed, and then frozen for subsequent analysis. After the 5-min rest interval, the collection reservoir was refilled with fresh solution. The 15-min current application and 5-min sampling procedure was repeated continuously over the duration of the experiment, 5 or more hours. Note that the electro-osmotic flux values were obtained over 15 min, and, hence, the flux values reported represent an average over that time period.

For the DC protocol, the polarity was constant; i.e., one skin site underwent anodal extraction and the other side cathodal extraction over the 4-h duration of the experiment. The AP (15) protocol was identical to the DC protocol, except that the polarity of the power supply was switched after the 15-min cycle and then switched back to the starting polarity after the subsequent 15-min cycle. In this protocol, the anode and cathode alternated from one site to the other during the course of the study. The AP (7.5) protocol was identical to the AP (15) protocol except the electrical polarity was reversed halfway through each 15-min cycle. In this protocol, each skin site had identical periods (7.5 min) of each polarity.

The extracts for all studies (diabetics and nondiabetics) were subsequently thawed and analyzed for glucose by high-performance liquid chromatography (HPLC) with pulsed amperometric detection according to a modification of a method developed by O'Shea et al.[13] The HPLC error was less than ±10% (relative standard deviation) and generally less than ±3% (relative standard deviation) as measured by repeated injection of standards throughout the chromatographic run. Verification of glucose peak identification was noted by selective disappearance of the glucose peak upon addition of glucose oxidase to the electroosmotic extract. The error in sample handling was estimated from the mass of buffer collected after each extraction period. Those results show that 6.4% error is introduced by the sample-handling procedure.

Written consent was obtained from all volunteers after they were informed of the nature and possible consequences of the study. The protocol was approved by an institutional review board. During the current application, subjects reported a mild tingling sensation, which diminished with time. Minor skin irritation, characterized by slight erythema and edema, was observed at the test site immediately after removal of the patches. In all cases, however, erythema and edema completely resolved in less than 1 week.

8.2.2 OPTIMIZATION STUDIES WITH SUBJECTS WITHOUT DIABETES

Optimization studies were performed on normal (those without diabetes) volunteer human subjects. Subjects fasted overnight before each evaluation. Each subject's blood glucose level was altered by oral ingestion of 75 g of glucose 1 h into the study. During the 5-min rest period between each extraction interval, blood glucose was measured by a standard finger prick (One Touch Basic, LifeScan, Milpitas, CA) method for comparison with extracted glucose flux.

To compare the electrical current application methods, AP (15) and DC protocols were performed simultaneously, one protocol on each arm, for each of 12 subjects, with the 0.45% unbuffered sodium chloride in water as the extraction solution.

Additionally, two subjects were compared DC to AP (15), one protocol on each arm, with the bicarbonate–saline mixture as the extraction solution. Finally, three subjects were compared with the bicarbonate solution in four successive testing sessions with the DC and AP (7.5) protocols performed simultaneously, one protocol on each arm for a total of 12 testing sessions.

8.2.3 HYPO- AND HYPERGLYCEMIC EVALUATIONS
WITH SUBJECTS WITH DIABETES

Three male and two female subjects from 22 to 58 years of age, diagnosed with either Type 1 or 2 diabetes mellitus for between 5 and 15 years, and a body weight within −30 to +50% of ideal as defined by the Metropolitan Life Insurance tables participated in the study. Subjects at medical risk or those with a skin disease on the forearms were excluded from the study. Subjects fasted for at least 8 h and omitted any insulin dose immediately prior to the study. To induce hyperglycemia, the subjects drank 100 g of glucose solution 1 h into the study. When the blood glucose reached 300 mg/dL, insulin (Humulin regular, Lilly, Indianapolis, IN) was administered intravenously (IV) to bring serum glucose to normal levels. To induce hypoglycemia, insulin was administered IV to achieve a target serum glucose of 40 to 60 mg/dL. Dextrose was then administered IV if the subject's serum glucose went below 40 mg/dL, or if the subject was below 60 mg/dL for longer than 60 min.

The investigation compared venous serum glucose measurements with glucose flux obtained by electroosmotic extraction. Blood samples were taken from an antecubital vein just before current was applied for the first time (0 time) and at the midpoint of each subsequent collection session (i.e., 7.5 min after initiation of current). The samples were sent to a clinical laboratory for serum glucose analysis using a Beckman CX-7 glucose analyzer. A drop of the each whole blood sample was also analyzed by the One Touch II or One Touch Basic meter to provide an immediate blood glucose measurement.

The current application method was AP (7.5) using the bicarbonate–saline extraction solution for all the subjects with diabetes. Three subjects were each tested in three successive sessions 1 week apart under the hyperglycemic protocol, and three subjects, one of whom was a repeat subject, were tested under the hypoglycemic protocol.

8.3 RESULTS AND DISCUSSION

8.3.1 OPTIMIZATION STUDIES

Figure 8.2a shows the results obtained for one subject without diabetes using the DC protocol (right arm) with unbuffered saline extraction solution. There was no apparent correlation between blood glucose and iontophoretic glucose flux. Results from 11 other subjects with the DC protocol were variable, with some subjects showing good correlation for collection at the anode, others at the cathode, and others, like the results shown here, exhibiting no correlation at either electrode.

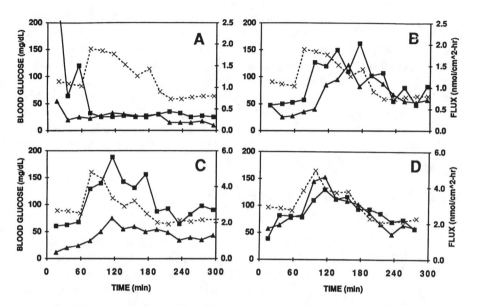

FIGURE 8.2 Blood glucose (-X-) vs. time compared with electroosmotic glucose flux (▲ anode or anode for first 7.5 min, ■ cathode or cathode for first 7.5 min) vs. time for a single human subject without diabetes. Conditions: (a) Right arm, DC, 0.9 mA, unbuffered saline extraction solution. (b) Same day as (a), but on left arm, AP (15), 0.9 mA, unbuffered saline extraction solution. (c) Different day as (a) and (b) AP, 0.9 mA, pH ~8.5 bicarbonate–saline extraction solution. (d) Different day, AP (7.5), 0.9 mA, pH ~8.5 bicarbonate–saline extraction solution.

Figure 8.2b shows data from the left arm of the same subject on the same day as in Figure 8.2a. Conditions were identical, except extraction was performed on the left arm with the AP (15) protocol. Note that the blood glucose profiles are identical for this comparison. The results show a striking improvement of the correlation using the AP (15) protocol. The enhanced response was observed for all 12 subjects evaluated, with all showing a statistically significant ($p = 0.05$) correlation between blood glucose and glucose flux. However, the AP (15) protocol led to an oscillatory response in some subjects, which led to poorer correlation. The oscillatory response (manifested in Figure 8.2b as a slight sawtooth pattern) is attributed to different glucose permeability at the two test sites as the cathode and anode alternated from site to site.

As shown by the results in Figure 8.2c, further improved correlation was achieved using the AP (15) protocol with bicarbonate–saline extraction solution. These results were obtained on the same subject as shown in Figure 8.2a and b (albeit on a separate testing session). The results show greater glucose flux at the cathode, consistent with electroosmotic extraction of glucose.[10] In particular, the bicarbonate–saline extraction solution (pH ~ 8.5) appears to have increased the negative charge of the skin, promoting sodium ion transport to the cathode and a concommitant increase in glucose flux.

These studies were extended to the AP (7.5) protocol wherein the current polarity was changed at 7.5 min into the 15-min extraction period, as shown in Figure 8.2d (again, the same subject without diabetes on a separate session). In this method, both extraction sites show similar glucose flux because both sites have had the same period (7.5 min) of cathodal and anodal extraction. Also, there is no oscillation in the flux values because the sites are kept constant in the AP (7.5) protocol, rather than switched as in the AP (15) protocol. These results and similar results from the two other subjects on four testing sessions each demonstrated a correlation between blood glucose and electroosmotically extracted glucose in subjects without diabetes using the AP (7.5) protocol with bicarbonate–saline.

8.3.2 HYPO- AND HYPERGLYCEMIC EVALUATONS WITH SUBJECTS WITH DIABETES

The optimized protocol using AP (7.5) with bicarbonate–saline extraction solution was used for studies on subjects with diabetes under hypo- and hyperglycemic blood glucose ranges. In Figure 8.3a and 3b, the flux values obtained at the two collection reservoirs were averaged for each time point, and the mean values are presented. A comparison of venous serum glucose and extracted glucose flux in two subjects with diabetes indicates that there is close tracking after an equilibration period in both the hypoglycemic (Figure 8.3a) and hyperglycemic (Figure 8.3b) range. This indicates that the extracted and serum measurements track over a glucose concentration range from 50 to 400 mg/dL. In four of five subjects, the extracted glucose flux traced serum values after the first 60 minutes, while in one subject tracking was not achieved until two hours into the study. This period is most likely due to the time required for skin hydration, equilibration of the skin with the extraction solution, or stabilization of the electrical properties of the skin.

Similar to the results obtained with subjects without diabetes, the results in Figure 8.3a and b show that the extracted glucose flux profile is shifted to a later time relative to the serum profile, suggesting a time lag between the two measurements. An estimate of the time lag was obtained from a series of linear regression analyses of serum glucose against glucose flux where each regression was determined with successive shifts in the sampling interval between the readings. In other words, the serum glucose values were analyzed vs. the extracted readings obtained during the overlapping time interval, and then with the values obtained one, two, or three sampling intervals later. In this way, the time lag yielding the largest correlation coefficient was determined as the "best fit." The best fit time lag ranged from zero to three sample periods, with an average of one sample interval for all evaluations; i.e., the serum value from the midpoint of one interval is correlated with the average flux of the next 20-min collection interval. This delay is caused by both the time required for the analyte to travel through the skin and the 20-min collection interval.

Results obtained for one subject on four separate days illustrates the tracking in successive measurements (Figure 8.4). The extracted glucose results shown in Figure 8.4 were all shifted forward by one collection period to match the time of the previous serum glucose measurement.

8.4 DISCUSSION AND CONCLUSIONS

A linear regression was performed with the data in Figure 8.4 for all times beyond 60 min. The results show an average correlation coefficient (r) of 0.91 for the four separate determinations. A similar analysis was performed for all 12 evaluations with the values for r, and the slope and intercept summarized in Table 8.1. The results show an average correlation coefficient of 0.89, demonstrating the close correlation between the extracted flux and plasma serum glucose values.

The results in Table 8.1 show that the intercept is generally close to zero, with 8 out of 12 studies showing a zero intercept ($p < 0.05$). Hence, to further simplify the analysis the glucose flux was divided by the serum glucose for each point, again assuming a one sample period time lag and omitting the data from the first hour. The results (Table 8.1) show that the ratio differed at most by a factor of two among all subjects tested with an average (standard error) of 4.12 (0.27) µm/h. It is interesting that the ratio obtained for the one-parameter fit shows less variability than the slope obtained with the two-parameter fit.

To be clinically useful, glucose measurements must be quantitatively reproducible and accurate. One criterion for establishing clinical accuracy is the error grid analysis.[14] The analysis divides the comparison between the reference serum glucose and the measured glucose (transdermal extraction in these experiments) into five zones. Values in zones A and B are clinically acceptable, whereas values in zones C, D, and E lead to clinically significant errors. We have developed a calibration method by dividing the serum glucose value during the third sample period (1 h, to allow the skin to equilibrate) by the extracted glucose flux taken one sample period later (to account for the time lag). This ratio was then used to calculate serum glucose from glucose flux for all subsequent measurements on that day. The calculated extracted glucose results for all subjects evaluated are shown in an error grid analysis in Figure 8.5. These results show that 136 of 140 data points (97%) are within the A and B region. Moreover, using a single-point calibration from day one for all subsequent data *on all days* for each subject resulted in 95% of the points within the A and B region. Equivalent error grid analysis results have been obtained for commercial whole blood glucose monitors.[15] These results demonstrate that the use of the single-point calibration produces quantitative values for glucose flux in the clinically acceptable region.

Another criterion for clinical accuracy is the mean absolute error between the reference and measured serum glucose value defined in these experiments by the following equation:

$$\text{Mean absolute error} = \text{Absolute value} \left[\frac{\text{Serum glucose} - \text{Extracted glucose}}{\text{Serum glucose}} \right]$$

The results obtained here show a mean absolute error of 12.9% for all measurements, a value comparable to currently available self-testing glucose monitors.[14,15] These results suggest that extracted glucose accurately and reproducibly reflects serum glucose values.

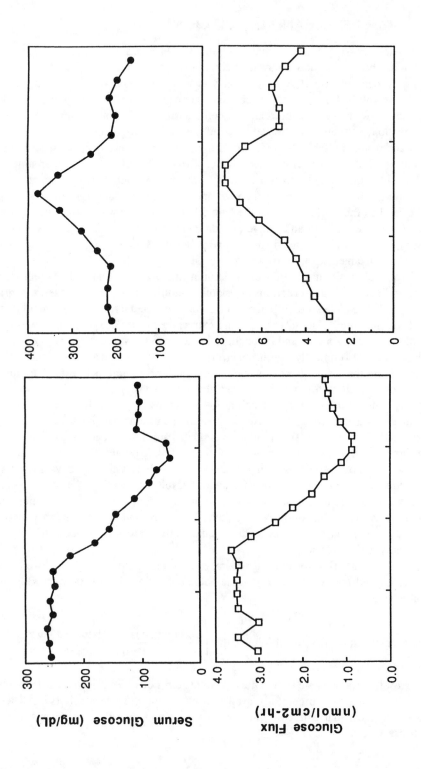

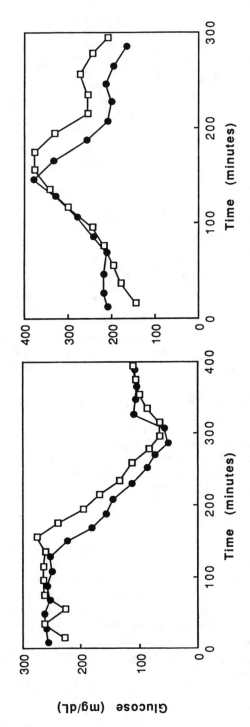

FIGURE 8.3 Serum glucose (●, top plot) and extracted glucose flux (□, middle plot) profiles. Extracted flux is reported as the average of the two sample chambers unless otherwise noted. The bottom plot shows a direct comparison of the glucose level calculated from the transdermally extracted glucose flux and the serum glucose. (a) Hypoglycemic response of Subject 4 (Type I): IV insulin was administered at 120 min and IV glucose was administered at 280 min. (b) Hyperglycemic response of Subject 2 (Type 2): oral glucose was administered at 60 min and IV insulin was administered at 120 min. (From Tamada, J. A., Bohannon, N. J. V., and Potts, R. O., *Nature Med.*, 1, 1198, 1995. With permission.)

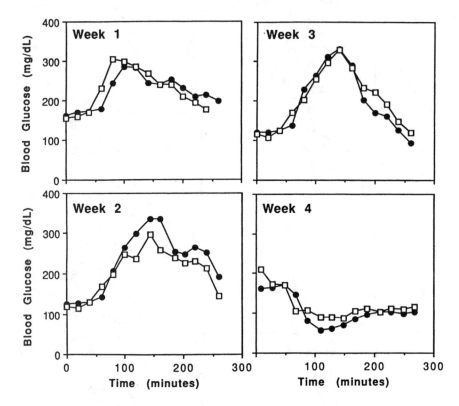

FIGURE 8.4 Comparison of serum glucose (●) and glucose calculated from the transdermally extracted glucose flux (□) from Subject 3 (Type 2) on four different days. The extraction data are uniformly shifted by an extraction period to match the time of the previous serum glucose measurement. Hyperglycemia was induced in sessions 1 to 3 and hypoglycemia on session 4. A single fingerprick calibration at the 1 h time point (as evidenced by the overlap of the two curves) was used to calculate equivalent serum glucose from the transdermally extracted glucose. (From Tamada, J. A., Bohannon, N. J. V., and Potts, R. O., *Nature Med.,* 1, 1198, 1995. With permission.)

In conclusion, correlation between serum glucose and extracted glucose was firmly established for five subjects under a variety of conditions. Quantitative measurement was possible through the use of a single-point calibration analysis. These results demonstrate a painless and bloodless method to extract glucose through the skin. Moreover, the correlation, error grid analysis, and mean absolute error results obtained were equivalent to those for commercial whole blood monitors.[14,15] Hence, the extraction technique potentially provides a noninvasive means to continuously monitor serum glucose in patients with diabetes, leading to the possibility for significantly enhanced health care.

TABLE 8.1
Relationship between Serum Glucose and Electroosmotic Flux

Subject		Number of Data Points	Linear Regression			Average Ratio of Flux to Serum Glucose (μm/h)
			r	Slope (μm/h)	Intercept (nmol/cm^2/h)	
			Hyperglycemic Protocol			
Subject 1	Week 1	12	0.98	5.55	−0.60[c]	5.14
	Week 2	12	0.89	3.15	1.36[c]	4.11
	Week 3[a]	12	0.93	4.20	0.59[c]	4.59
Subject 2	Week 1[b]	9	0.67	3.43	2.26[c]	4.74
	Week 2[a,b]	9	0.98	2.09	0.91	3.10
	Week 3[a,b]	9	0.92	1.78	2.78	3.68
Subject 3	Week 1	12	0.79	6.28	−0.96[c]	5.37
	Week 2	12	0.93	3.34	1.37[c]	4.38
	Week 3	12	0.96	2.49	0.84[c]	3.30
			Hypoglycemic Protocol			
Subject 3[a]		12	0.83	1.81	1.01	3.70
Subject 4		17	0.99	2.46	0.02[c]	2.48
Subject 5		12	0.96	2.26	1.38	4.79
AVERAGE			**0.89**	**3.24**	**0.91**	**4.12**

Note: Regressions and ratios were calculated using an equilibration period and a one sample period time lag.

[a] Data from a single collection chamber rather than average of two chambers.
[b] Subject required 2-h equilibration period.
[c] Intercept not significantly different from zero ($p = 0.05$).

Source: Tamada, J. A., Bohannon, N. J. V., and Potts, R. O., *Nature Med.*, 1, 1198 (1995). With permission.

ACKNOWLEDGEMENTS

The authors would like to thank Nooshin Azimi, Kathleen Comyns, Lewis Leung, Kamran Rafii, Mark Burns, Michael Sekera, and Gabriel Chan for their technical support of this work. Richard Guy provided invaluable scientific insight into these studies.

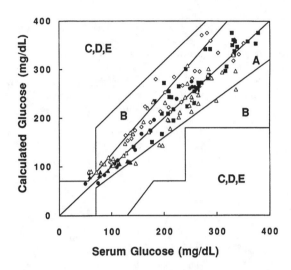

FIGURE 8.5 Error grid analysis for all five subjects, 12 experiments ($n = 140$) with calculations as described in the text and in Table 8.1. Subject 1 (■), Subject 2 (◊), Subject 3 (△), Subject 4 (●), Subject 5 (▲). (From Tamada, J. A., Bohannon, N. J. V., and Potts, R. O., *Nature Med.*, 1, 1198, 1995. With permission.)

REFERENCES

1. The Diabetes Control and Complications Trial Research Group, The effect of intensive treatment of diabetes on the development and progression of long-term complications in insulin-dependent diabetes mellitus, *N. Engl. J. Med.*, 329, 977 (1993).
2. Meyerhoff, C., Bischof, F., Sternberg, F., Zier, H., and Pfeiffer, E. F., On line continuous monitoring of subcutaneous tissue glucose in men by combining portable glucosensor with microdialysis, *Diabetologia*, 35, 1087 (1992).
3. Moatti-Sirat, D., Capron, F., Poitout, V., Reach, G., Bindra, D. S., Zhang, Y., Wilson, G. S., and Thevenot, D. R., Towards continuous glucose monitoring: *in vivo* evaluation of a miniaturized glucose sensor implanted for several days in rat subcutaneous tissue, *Diabetologia*, 35, 224 (1992).
4. Reach, G. and Wilson, G., Can continuous glucose monitoring be used for the treatment of diabetes? *Anal. Chem.*, 64, 381 (1992).
5. Reach, G., Continuous glucose monitoring with a subcutaneous sensor. Rationale, requirements and achievements, and prospectives, in *The Diabetes Annual*, Alberti, K. G. M. M. and Home, P. D., Eds., Elsevier, New York (1993), p. 332.
6. Glikfeld, P., Hinz, R. S., and Guy, R. H., Noninvasive sampling of biological fluids by iontophoresis, *Pharm. Res.*, 6, 988 (1989).
7. Rao, G., Glikfeld, P., Guy, R., H., Reverse iontophoresis: development of a noninvasive approach for glucose monitoring, *Pharm. Res.*, 10, 1751 (1993).
8. Rao, G., Tamada, J., Azimi N., Leung, L., Plantew, P., Potts, R. O., Glikfeld, P., LaCourse, W. R., and Guy, R. H., Iontophoretic and noninvasive glucose monitoring, in *Proc. Int. Symp. Controlled Release Bioact. Mater.*, Vol. 21, Controlled Release Society, Deerfield, IL (1994), p. 13.

9. Green, P. G., Flanagan, M., Shroot, B., and Guy, R. H., Iontophoretic drug delivery, in *Pharmaceutical Skin Penetration Enhancement,* Vol. 59, Walters, K. A. and Hadgraft, J., Eds., Marcel Dekker, New York (1993), p. 311.

10. Pikal, M. J. and Shah, S., Transport mechanisms in iontophoresis. III. An experimental study of the contributions of electroosmotic flow and permeability change in transport of low and high molecular weight solutes, *Pharm. Res.,* **7**, 222 (1990).

11. Tamada, J. A., Bohannon, N. J. V., and Potts, R. O, Measurement of glucose in diabetic subjects using noninvasive transdermal extraction, *Nature Med.,* 1, 1198 (1995).

12. Tamada, J. A., Azimi, N. T., Leung, L., Plante, P., and Potts, R. O., Correlation of blood glucose with iontophoretic glucose flux in human subjects for glucose monitoring, in *Proc. Int. Symp. Control. Release of Bioact. Mater.,* Vol. 22, Controlled Release Society, Deerfield, IL (1995), p. 129.

13. O'Shea, T. J., Lunte, S. M., and LaCourse, W. R., Detection of carbohydrates by capillary electrophoresis with pulsed amperometric detection, *Anal. Chem.,* 64, 381 (1992).

14. Clarke, W. L., Cox, D. C., Conder-Frederick, L. A., Carter, W., Pohl, S. L., Evaluating clinical accuracy of systems for self-monitoring of blood glucose, *Diabetes Care,* 10, 622 (1987)

15. Karbadi, U. M., O'Connell, K. M., Johnson, J., and Karbadi, M., The effect of recurrent practice at home on the acceptability of capillary blood glucose readings, *Diabetes Care,* 17, 1110 (1994).

9 Medtronic SynchroMed Infusion System

Kenneth T. Heruth

CONTENTS

9.1 INTRODUCTION

Implantable infusion pumps have been in use since 1976. In that time period, they have become an important therapeutic tool. Implantable infusion pumps have several advantages over alternative infusion methods: they require virtually no patient inter-action, reduce the potential for infection, need to be refilled infrequently which requires less medical care, and can deliver drugs directly to an organ that is not easily accessed, e.g., to the brain or spinal cord, which reduces the amount of drug that is required to be effective and reduces side effects.

The Medtronic SynchroMed® system is a completely implantable infusion sys-tem which is also programmable. The infusion rate can be noninvasively adjusted to compensate for changing requirements, such as an increase in daily medication. Infusion rate can also be programmed to change automatically during the day to accommodate different requirements, e.g., during periods of sleep compared with periods of wakefulness. An electromechanical pump accurately infuses drugs over a wide range of infusion rates.

Medtronic, Inc. was founded in 1949 to repair medical equipment for hospitals. Subsequently, Medtronic became a pioneer in the development of battery-powered heart pacemakers, first external, then implantable devices. Today, Medtronic's prod-ucts include bradycardia pacemakers, implantable defibrillators, heart valves, surgi-cal blood pumps and blood oxygenators, percutaneous transluminal arterial catheters and guiding catheters, and implantable spinal cord stimulators. The technology required to develop this wide range of products has been applied to the SynchroMed implantable infusion system. Electronic, software, mechanical, and biomaterials expertise, as well as expertise in developing implantable devices and conducting

0-8493-7681-5/98/$0.00+$.50
© 1998 by CRC Press LLC

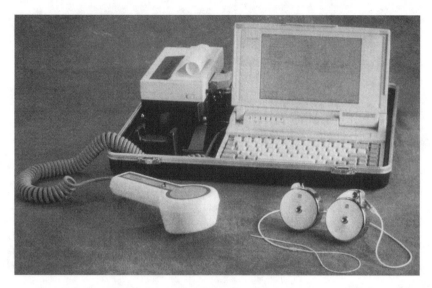

FIGURE 9.1   SynchroMed system components.

complex clinical trials have all contributed to the development of this sophisticated system. The first SynchroMed pump was implanted in 1982. After extensive clinical trials, it was commercially released in the U.S. for cancer chemotherapy in 1987. More recently, it has been commercially released for management of malignant and nonmalignant pain, and for management of chronic intractable spasticity of spinal cord origin.

9.2   DESCRIPTION OF SYSTEM

The SynchroMed system consists of an implantable infusion pump, an external programmer, a variety of implantable infusion catheters, and surgical accessories, as shown in Figure 9.1. All of these components contribute to the performance of the system.

The SynchroMed pump is a completely implantable device. It can be refilled percutaneously, and can be interrogated and programmed using an external programmer.

The pump is enclosed in a cylindrical titanium case approximately 25 mm thick and 75 mm in diameter. Titanium is a biocompatible material that has been used for many years to manufacture implantable devices, such as pacemakers and orthopedic implants. Inside the titanium case are a drug reservoir, a battery, an electromechanical pump, and an electronic control circuit. A diagram of the internal components is shown in Figure 9.2.

The implantable SynchroMed pump is powered by a lithium battery, similar to batteries used in other implantable medical devices. The battery has an expected life of 36 to 48 months, depending on the fluid infusion rate.

A titanium bellows provides a storage reservoir for the drug. The bellows collapses as drug is withdrawn. The leaves of the bellows are shaped to conform to

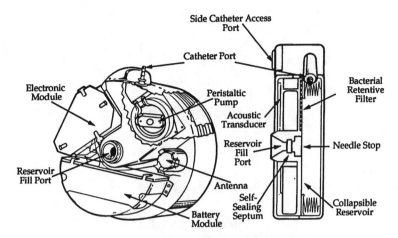

FIGURE 9.2   SynchroMed pump internal components.

each other, so that the amount of trapped fluid is minimized. For accurate infusion, it is necessary to maintain a constant reservoir pressure. To do so, a fluid in equilibruim between liquid and vapor phases is used to compensate for changes in reservoir volume.

The reservoir can be accessed for refilling by percutaneously puncturing a self-sealing septum with a noncoring hypodermic needle. Syringes are used to withdraw any remaining fluid from the reservoir and to inject fresh drug into the reservoir. Recently, a shutoff valve has been built into the refill column to prevent overfilling the reservoir. If the reservoir were overfilled, a high reservoir pressure would be created and infusion accuracy could be affected.

A filter with 0.22 μm pore size is placed at the outlet of the reservoir. Fluid passes through the filter as it is drawn from the reservoir into the pump. The filter will screen out any bacteria or particles that may have entered the reservoir.

A peristaltic, or roller pump, controls infusion of the fluid. The pump meters the fluid through a silicone tube to the outlet of the SynchroMed. The peristaltic pump will deliver the programmed amount over a wide variety of conditions. For example, for some therapies, the drug is delivered into the cerebrospinal fluid (CSF) which is at a very low pressure. For other therapies, the drug is infused into the arterial system, which has a much higher, pulsatile, pressure. Infusion rate can also potentially be affected by altitude, patient body temperature, and fluid viscosity. However, the SynchroMed pump will accurately deliver fluid over all expected conditions.

The peristaltic pump is driven by a stepper motor. Infusion rate is controlled by the frequency of pulses from the electronic control module. For safety, the infusion rate has a mechanical limit as well as a limit in the electronic control; the motor will not respond to very rapid pulse rates. As an additional safety mechanism, on/off pulses of alternating polarity are required to drive the stepper motor. If the electronic control system would fail in an "on" state, the pump will not rotate.

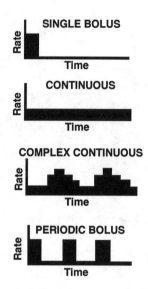

FIGURE 9.3   Infusion modes.

A microcomputer-based hybrid electronic circuit controls the SynchroMed pump. It sends pulses to the pump stepper motor based on the programmed infusion requirements. An antenna allows communication with the external programmer using radio frequency (RF) signals. An implanted SynchroMed can be reprogrammed for different infusion modes, infusion rates, or reservoir volume. The status of these variables, as well as the status of alarm conditions, can also be interrogated using the programmer.

The hybrid control circuit can also activate an audible indicator if alarm conditions occur, including a reservoir volume below a programmable level, battery near depletion, or corrupted program data.

The infusion rate can be programmed to rates between 0.1 and 21 ml/day. The control circuit can also be programmed to alter the infusion at a preset time. Four infusion modes are available, as illustrated in Figure 9.3. The infusion modes include

- *Bolus* — Infuses a programmed amount, then returns to the previous infusion mode;
- *Simple Continuous* — Infuses fluid at a constant rate;
- *Complex Continuous* — Allows setting up to ten distinct infusion rates and time intervals (at the end of a complete pattern, the control circuit will return to the beginning and repeat the program);
- *Bolus-Delay* — infuses fluid in periodic boluses (the amount and time interval for each bolus can be programmed).

An optional catheter access port is available for the SynchroMed pump. The access port is attached to the side of the SynchroMed, as seen in Figure 9.2. This

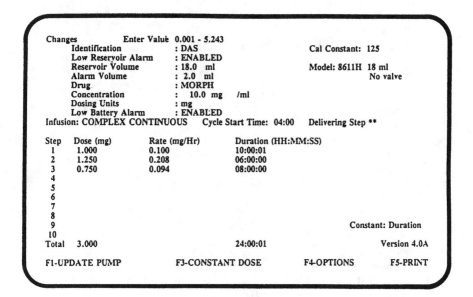

FIGURE 9.4 Programmer screen.

allows infusion of a fluid, such as a radiopaque marker or a different drug, directly into the catheter without passing through the pump. The access port septum is protected by a screen. The screen prevents a 22-gauge needle, which is normally used to refill the pump reservoir, from penetrating the access port septum. A special 25-gauge needle is required to puncture the access port septum.

The programmer is based on a laptop computer. The computer has been interfaced to a special RF telemetry head for communication with implanted SynchroMed pumps. The computer and telemetry head are packaged, along with a printer, in a portable carrying case. Programmers are used in the operating room, hospital room, clinic, and in a patient's home for refill procedures. The programmer software is designed to make programming straightforward. Programming is performed in terms that are familiar to the clinician; e.g., some drugs are typically prescribed in milligram per day, while others are prescribed in micrograms per day per kilogram of body weight. The programmer will also print information for the patient's record, such as patient identification and drug name. All information is displayed simultaneously on a single screen. A sample screen is shown in Figure 9.4.

Drug is routed from the pump to the site of delivery through a catheter. The SynchroMed is a flexible system that can be used to deliver chronically different types of drugs. Catheters have been developed to deliver drugs into body sites such as the venous and arterial systems, the epidural or intrathecal space of the spine, the brain, and the peritoneal cavity.

Surgical accessories have been developed to aid the surgical implant procedure. These include anchors for the pump and catheter, tunneling devices, and catheter guide wires. Accessory kits are also available for the refill procedure and to inject

TABLE 9.1
Drugs Compatible with the SynchroMed System

Drug	Application	Stability, days
Pre-Market Approved[a]		
Baclofen	Spasticity	90
Clindamycin	Osteomyolitis	7
Doxorubicin (Adriamycin)	Cancer chemotherapy	14
Floxuridine (FUDR)	Cancer chemotherapy	28
Morphine sulfate PF	Pain Control	90
Vinblastine (Velban)	Cancer chemotherapy	28
Tested[b]		
Cisplatin	Cancer chemotherapy	7
Dobutamine	Congestive heart failure	7
Methotrexate	Cancer chemotherapy	28
Bleomycin	Cancer chemotherapy	3
Flourouracil	Cancer chemotherapy	28
Heparin	Anticoagulant	28
Naloxone	Analgesic	28
Bethanechol	Alzheimer's disease	42
Thyrotropin-releasing hormone	Amyotrophic lateral sclerosis	28
Mitoxantrone	Cancer chemotherapy	28
Interferon α-2A: α-2B	Cancer chemotherapy	7
Octreotide[c]	Pain control	28
Neostigmine	Alzheimer's disease	28
Insulin GH	Diabetes	28
Insulin Humulin II	Diabetes	28

[a] Pre-market approved in the U.S.
[b] Tested and found compatible.
[c] Requires pH adjustment to 6.5.

through the catheter access port. In addition to needles and syringes, the kits include a template to assist in locating the septum.

The implantable components must be made from materials that are biocompatible and biostable when implanted within the body for long periods of time. They must also be compatible and stable with any drugs that will be used in the system. The SynchroMed system is designed with materials that have a long history of biocompatibility. Each drug intended for use in the system is tested for compatibility with the SynchroMed fluid pathway. A list of drugs that have been tested for compatibility with the SynchroMed system is shown in Table 9.1. It should be noted from Table 9.1 that the inherent stability of some drugs may require more frequent refill intervals.

9.3   SURGICAL PROCEDURES

The SynchroMed system is surgically implanted in the proper site in the body. The time required for the procedure depends on the placement of the catheter, but typically takes about 1 h.

The first step in implanting the system is placing the catheter. Surgical techniques have been developed to place catheters in the arterial system, the intrathecal or epidural space, and the brain. These standard techniques are used to place the SynchroMed catheters. Since the SynchroMed catheters are left in place long term, the entry site must be carefully sealed and the catheter securely anchored. After all suturing and anchoring, it is verified that the catheter lumen is still patent. The catheter is filled with water or saline, to displace air from the catheter.

The pump is usually implanted in the abdomen, but may be implanted in the pectoral region for some applications. The pump is typically implanted about 2.5 cm deep. This protects the pump, but makes it accessible for refilling. An incision is made at the pump site, then a subcutaneous pocket is formed. The pocket is made large enough to accept the pump, with a tight fit. The catheter is then tunneled subcutaneously from its entry site to the pump pocket, using a tunneling rod or hollow tube.

The pump is shipped from the factory with sterile water in the reservoir. In preparation for implantation, the water is replaced with drug. To perform the refill procedure, the pump is warmed to body temperature to bring the reservoir to its normal pressure. The pump is removed from its package in the sterile field and placed in a basin of warmed sterile water. Before refilling, a small bolus is programmed into the pump to purge any air out of the fluid pathway. The pump is observed to ensure that fluid is leaving the catheter port. A noncoring needle is inserted into the reservoir septum. The water is removed from the reservoir and replaced with drug. The pump is again programmed, to enter the appropriate drug information and reservoir volume into the pump control circuit and to set the pump at an appropriate infusion rate.

The pump is connected to the catheter, and a suture tied over the connector. The pump is then slid into the pocket and sutured to the underlying fascia. To assist in suturing the pump, it can be enclosed in a mesh pouch, or it can be ordered with optional metal suture loops. To complete the procedure, incisions at the pump pocket and at the catheter entry site are sutured closed.

Subsequent refill procedures can be performed whenever necessary. The programmer is first used to determine the present status of the pump. The patient's skin over the pump site is then cleaned. A noncoring needle is attached to an extension set with a shutoff device. With the extension set blocked, the noncoring needle is inserted into the septum. An empty syringe is connected to the extension set; the extension set is opened and all fluid is withdrawn from the reservoir. The extension set is again blocked to prevent any air from entering the reservoir. The syringe containing old drug is removed, and a syringe with the fresh drug is connected. The extension set is opened, and the fresh drug is injected into the septum. Finally, the programmer is used to enter the new drug information into the control circuit, and to alter the infusion mode or rate if desired.

9.4   CLINICAL EXPERIENCE

The SynchroMed system is a tool that can be used by physicians to deliver drugs chronically. The drug provides the therapy, rather than the device. The purpose of the SynchroMed system is to deliver the desired drug to the proper location in the body. The SynchroMed system has been used clinically for several different applications. Some examples are described below.

The SynchroMed system has been used to infuse chemotherapeutic agents for treatment of cancer. As an example, floxuridine (FUDR) has been infused into the hepatic artery to treat metastatic gastrointestinal carcinoma.[1] The implantable infusion system delivers the drug directly to the site of the tumor. The patient receives the drug over several days, and can be ambulatory the entire time. The programmable features of the SynchroMed can be used to match the infusion rate to the periodic susceptibility of the malignant cells to reduce the amount of FUDR that is required for effectiveness.

Severe, chronic pain can be caused by diseases such as cancer, or by injury to nerves or body tissue. In most cases, adequate relief can be obtained through exercise, oral medication, or surgical procedure. However, some patients do not respond to these therapies. For those patients, the SynchroMed system can be used to infuse opiates or other analgesics directly to the spinal cord.[2-4] The medication is delivered into the CSF surrounding the spinal cord, where it interrupts pain signals that are transmitted to the brain. This minimizes the required amount of drug and minimizes side effects.

Spinal cord injury, multiple sclerosis, and cerebral palsy can cause severe, repeated spasms or rigidity in legs and arms. Relief can usually be obtained with oral medication. However, some people do not respond to the oral medication, or have unacceptable side effects. For these patients, the SynchroMed system is used to infuse baclofen, an antispastic agent, directly into the CSF surrounding the spinal cord.[5-8] By infusing baclofen close to its site of action, the effective dose is reduced relative to oral doses, and the drug side effects are minimized.

Other potential therapies for the SynchroMed system are in an early evaluation stage. These include treatment of neurological diseases such as Alzheimer's disease, Parkinson's disease, and amyotrophic lateral sclerosis (Lou Gehrig's disease).

9.5   CONCLUSION

The SynchroMed system is a commercially released system that has been implanted in thousands of patients. It has proved to be a safe and effective tool in treating chronic, intractable medical conditions. Drug delivery directly to the targeted organ and external programmability have provided improved drug efficacy and better cost-effectiveness than alternative infusion technologies. In the future, the SynchroMed system will be utilized for additional therapies that require accurate, controllable drug infusion.

REFERENCES

1. Roemeling, R. V. and Hrushesky, W. J. M., Circadian pattern of continuous FUDR infusion reduces toxicity, in *Advances in Chronobiology, Part B*, Alan R. Liss, New York, 1987, 357–373.
2. Hasenbusch, S. J. et al., Constant infusion of morphine for intractable cancer pain using an implanted pump, *J. Neurosurgery,* 73, 405–409, 1990.
3. Portenoy, R. K., Chronic opioid therapy in nonmalignant pain, *J. Pain Symptom Manage.,* 5(1) (Suppl.), February, 1990.
4. Krames, E. S., Intrathecal infusional therapies for intractable pain: patient management guidelines, *J. Pain Symptom Manage.,* 8(1), 36–46, 1993.
5. Penn, R. D. et al., Intrathecal baclofen for severe spinal spasticity, *N. Engl. J. Med.,* 320, 1517–1521, 1989.
6. Lazorthes, Y. et al., Chronic intrathecal baclofen administration for control of severe spasticity, *J. Neurosurgery,* 72, 393–402, 1990.
7. Coffey, R. J. et al., Intrathecal baclofen for intractable spasticity of spinal origin: results of a long-term multicenter study, *J. Neurosurgery,* 78, 226–232, 1993.
8. Albright, A. L. et al., Continuous intrathecal baclofen infusion for spasticity of cerebral origin, *J. Am. Med. Assoc.,* 270(20), 2475–2477, 1993.

10 Electroporation

Mark R. Prausnitz

CONTENTS

10.1 INTRODUCTION

Controlled drug delivery is generally achieved by manipulating the properties of drugs and/or drug delivery devices or carriers. However, once a drug leaves its carrier (whether it is a syringe, transdermal patch, or microsphere), direct control of drug transport through the body's tissues is generally not possible. If one were able to control the transport properties of biological barriers within the body, then drug delivery could be more completely controlled, including both the release of the drug from a carrier as well as drug transport through tissues to the therapeutic target. Electroporation of biological barriers makes this type of control a possibility.

Electroporation has been applied to drug delivery primarily in three areas. The first application involves loading drug into cells which then act as biocompatible carriers. Second, approaches to enhancing cancer chemotherapy have been explored, where locally increased permeability of tumors caused by electroporation can lead to greatly enhanced therapy with fewer side effects, as seen *in vivo* and in the clinic. Finally, electroporation of skin has been shown to occur and increase transdermal transport of molecules by orders of magnitude, as demonstrated through electrical, molecular flux, and microscopy studies *in vitro*.

10.2   BACKGROUND OF ELECTROPORATION

Electroporation involves the creation of transient aqueous pathways in lipid bilayer membranes by the application of a short electric field pulse.[1-5] Permeability and electrical conductance of lipid bilayers are rapidly increased by many orders of magnitude, where membrane changes can be reversible or irreversible. Electroporation occurs when the transmembrane voltage reaches on the order of 1 V for electric field pulses typically of 10 μs to 10 ms in duration. Electroporation is known to occur in metabolically inactive systems, such as black lipid membranes[6] and red blood cell ghosts,[7,8] as well as in living cells[1,3] and tissues.[4,9] While other terms, such as electropermeabilization,[4] are also used in the literature, we have followed the most common practice and refer to this phenomenon as electroporation.[1-3,5]

Electrical studies have shown that membrane resistance can drop orders of magnitude on a timescale of microseconds or faster due to electroporation.[10-12] Typically, upon applying a pulse, the membrane charges and initially remains stable (Figure 10.1). Then, the membrane becomes unstable and electroporation occurs, resulting in dramatically reduced membrane resistance. These changes in membrane electrical properties can be reversible or irreversible, depending largely on pulse parameters and membrane geometry.

Molecular transport across membranes also increases during electroporation. As shown in Figure 10.2, large numbers of macromolecules, such as bovine serum albumin (BSA), can be introduced into cells. Gene transfection can be accomplished when DNA is transported across cell membranes and incorporated into the genetic material of a cell, a technique routinely used in molecular biology.[1,3]

The mechanism of transport caused by electroporation is expected to involve diffusion and/or electrically driven transport (Figure 10.3). During a pulse, transport has been shown to occur by electrophoresis and/or electroosmosis (Figure 10.3A and B), depending on the experimental system.[7,13,14] For small compounds (e.g., $M_r <$ 1000 Da), significant transport can also occur by diffusion after a pulse due to long-lived changes in membrane permeability (Figure 10.3C and D). Postpulse transport of macromolecules is generally much slower.

Although studied mostly in planar bilayer and isolated cell systems, electroporation has also been demonstrated in cells part of monolayers[15,16] and in tissues, including retinal explants,[17] islets of Langerhans,[18,19] rice,[20] and maize[21] tissues, in skeletal muscle,[22] in a number of different tumors,[23-27] and in the dermis[28] and stratum corneum[29-33] of the skin.

The dramatic and often-reversible changes in membrane properties associated with electroporation have been explained with models involving transient creation of aqueous pathways, or "pores," across the lipid bilayer.[34-37] However, direct evidence

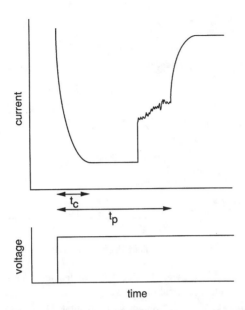

FIGURE 10.1   General features of the events occurring during electroporation of a planar bilayer membrane. During the application of a square-wave voltage pulse (lower graph), the current (upper graph) is initially large due to charging of the membrane. After a characteristic charging time, t_c, the current is approximately constant until it rapidly surges and then fluctuates, believed to be caused by membrane instability. Upon electroporation of the membrane, after a characteristic poration time, t_p, the current rapidly rises due to the creation of aqueous pathways across the membrane. In isolated planar bilayer membranes, electroporation often results in permanent membrane rupture. However, in spherical membranes, cells, and tissues, electroporation is usually partially or fully reversible. (From Abidor, I. G. et al., *Bioelectrochem. Bioenerget.*, 104, 37, 1979. With permission.)

(i.e., visualization) for these pores has not been reported, primarily because electropores are believed to be small (<10 nm), sparse (<0.1% of surface area), and generally short-lived (microseconds to seconds), making their capture by any form of microscopy extremely difficult.[38]

10.3   APPLICATIONS IN DRUG DELIVERY

10.3.1   LOADING OF CELLS AS DRUG CARRIERS

For controlled release of drug from an environment protected from the degradative enzymes of the body, drugs have been encapsulated in carrier systems, such as microspheres and liposomes.[39-41] Problems associated with these approaches can include inactivation of drug during the encapsulation process and poor biocompatibility of the carrier.

Electroporation has been used to load a variety of different molecules into red blood cell ghosts, which can act as drug carriers. Ghost-encapsulated compounds

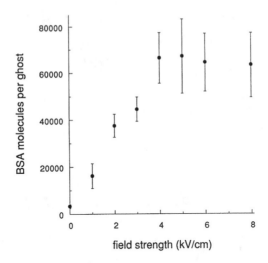

FIGURE 10.2   Uptake of fluorescein-labeled BSA molecules by erythrocyte ghosts as a function of pulse magnitude. Spherical ghosts were suspended in a solution containing BSA and exposed to a single exponential-decay pulse (decay time constant, $\tau = 1$ to 2 ms). Initially, uptake of exogenous BSA increased with field strength, while above approximately 4 kV/cm a plateau in uptake is observed. The BSA concentration inside the ghosts in the high-voltage plateau region is estimated to be only 7% of the extracellular concentration (10^{-5} M). Models of electroporation which account for the dynamic, voltage-dependent behavior of the pore population can explain this subequilibrium plateau.[102] This figure includes data from on the order of 10^6 individual ghosts measured by flow cytometry. Standard error bars are shown. (From Prausnitz, M. R. et al., *Biophys. J.*, 65, 414, 1993. With permission.)

include proteins and enzymes which retain their biological activity.[42] To test the *in vivo* application of this approach, intact murine red blood cells were loaded by electroporation with a model drug, (^{14}C)-sucrose, which was later released *in vivo* in a mouse (Figure 10.4).[43] This carrier system was biologically inert and maintained a constant (^{14}C)-sucrose plasma concentration over the 30-day period of the experiment. While encapsulation by electroporation is a gentle process which can yield biologically active drug inside biocompatible carriers, limitations of the approach include biohazards associated with the likely use of human blood, lack of control over release rates, and very slow release rates for encapsulated macromolecules.

Another application of electroporation for controlled drug delivery involves targeting drug delivery to leukocytes. Because the voltage drop across a cell is a function of the cell diameter, electroporation of large cells occurs at lower bulk field strengths than that of small cells.[1,3] By taking advantage of this targeting mechanism, whole blood was exposed to electroporation pulses which permeabilized leukocytes (which are generally larger than erythrocytes), but left erythrocytes unaffected (i.e., they did not undergo hemolysis).[44] This approach could be used to deliver drugs selectively to leukocytes, which could act as drug carriers targeted to the immune system.

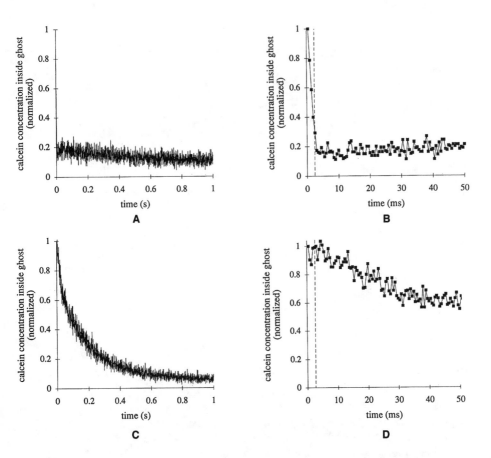

FIGURE 10.3 Normalized calcein concentration inside individual calcein-loaded erythrocyte ghosts during and after single exponential decay electric field pulses ($E = 2.5$ kV/cm; $\tau = 2.5 \pm 1$ ms), measured with a fluorescence microscope photometer with millisecond time resolution. In each case, the ghost was completely emptied of calcein, but over different timescales. (A and B) Most efflux occurred during the pulse, suggesting transport primarily by electrophoresis and/or electro-osmosis. (C and D) Most efflux occurred after the pulse, suggesting transport primarily by diffusion across a permeabilized membrane. Each pair of graphs (e.g., A and B) contains the same data shown on different timescales. The dashed lines indicate the time constant, τ, of the pulse. (From Prausnitz, M. R. et al., *Biophys. J.*, 68, 1864, 1995. With permission.)

10.3.2 PERMEABILIZATION OF TUMORS
FOR ENHANCED CHEMOTHERAPY

The success of cancer chemotherapy is often limited by the inability of therapeutic agents to reach their targets inside tumors.[45] Moreover, side effects from drugs reaching unintended targets elsewhere in the body are also a significant problem.

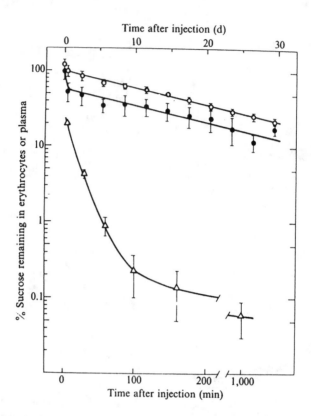

FIGURE 10.4   Elimination of sucrose from the circulation of mice. Murine erythrocytes were loaded with (^{14}C)-sucrose by electroporation and subsequently allowed to reseal. Sucrose entrapped in fully resealed erythrocytes (○), in partially resealed erythrocytes (●), or free in solution (△) was injected into AKR/J female mice. While free sucrose was eliminated within hours, entrapped sucrose was eliminated over a half-life of about 2 weeks, corresponding to the known half-life of mouse erythrocytes. Over the 30-day period of the experiment, the sucrose plasma concentration in the presence of loaded erythrocytes was approximately constant and equal to about 0.1% of the concentration inside the loaded erythrocytes. Standard deviation bars are shown. (From Kinosita, K. and Tsong, T. Y., *Nature*, 272, 258, 1978. With permission.)

To address both of these issues, electroporation of tumors has been used to deliver drug selectively to tumors, thereby increasing drug effectiveness and reducing side effects.[23-27] Work has been performed *in vitro*, *in vivo*, and clinically using the drug bleomycin.

10.3.2.1   *In Vitro*

Electroporation *in vitro* of DC-3F cells, a spontaneously transformed Chinese hamster lung fibroblast line, resulted in increased uptake of bleomycin and consequent drug-induced cell death.[46,47] On average, 400 bleomycin molecules needed to be transported inside each cell to kill it.[47] Because electroporation enhanced transport

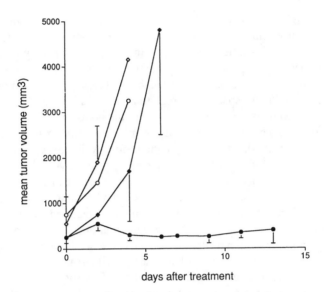

FIGURE 10.5 Tumor growth in mice following different electrical and pharmacological treatments. B16 melanomas in the flanks of C57B1/6 mice received no treatment (◊), or were treated with drug only (○), electric pulses only (♦), or both drug and electric pulses (●). Tumors treated with both drug (500 μg bleomycin, intramuscular injection) and electric pulses (8 pulses applied across the tumors at 1000 V, 100 μs, 1 pulse/s) showed 4 complete regressions and 1 cure out of 11 treated mice. Other treatment protocols resulted in no regression or cures. Because bleomycin crosses cell membranes very poorly, permeabilization of tumors by electroporation pulses is expected to increase bleomycin uptake and thereby increase its therapeutic effect. (From Mir, L. M. et al., *Eur. J. Cancer*, 27, 68, 1991. With permission.)

of drug across cell membranes, the externally applied bleomycin dose required for cell death was up to 10,000 times smaller with electroporation than without.[47] In contrast, electroporation enhanced drug effectiveness only three- to fivefold for lipophilic drugs which could more easily cross cell membranes, suggesting that the mechanism of bleomycin enhancement was related to increased transmembrane transport.[46] Moreover, the effects of melphalan on cells is normally controlled by leucine concentration, since melphalan enters cells via leucine transporters. However, leucine concentration did not influence the effects of melphalan on electroporated cells, suggesting that leucine transporters did not control transport because electroporation created new transmembrane pathways.[46]

10.3.2.2 *In Vivo*

Treatment *in vivo* has been performed on a number of different types of tumors in mouse, rat, and rabbit models.[4,9] In each of the studies, treatment with either bleomycin (by intramuscular or intravenous injection) or electric pulses (applied at the site of the tumor) alone did not have significant effects on tumor size. However, the combination of bleomycin and electroporation resulted in significant reduction in tumor size and prolongation of animal life (Figure 10.5).[23-25,27,48-52] For example, in one study involving spontaneous mammary tumors in mice, all 38 of the animals treated with electrochemotherapy showed at least partial regression, while 23 showed complete regression, 3 of which were cures.[49] In electrochemotherapy studies, typical electrical protocols have involved application of 1 to 8 square-wave or exponential-decay pulses of 600 to 10,000 V in strength and 0.1 to 7 ms in duration across electrodes of 2 to 25 mm spacing.[53] Local transient edema, superficial skin scabs, and local tissue necrosis can be associated with the protocol.[25,48]

To establish whether or not the mechanism of this therapy involved increased drug uptake by tumors due to electroporation, bleomycin concentration was measured throughout the body 3 days after treatment of mice *in vivo*.[52] Drug concentration in the treated tumors was approximately four times greater in mice that had received electric pulses than those that had not. In all other tissues, drug concentration was the same independent of whether or not tumors had received electrical treatment. This indicates that drug was targeted by electroporation to the site of the tumors. Further mechanistic insight may also come from experiments which have shown that the combination of bleomycin electrochemotherapy with treatment with interleukin-2 further increases the number of animals cured.[54-56] This suggests that the immune system plays a role in tumor cell death associated with electrochemotherapy.

As expected for electroporation, the success of electrochemotherapy treatment depends strongly on pulse voltage and duration. In general, tumoricidal effects are seen above a minimum threshold voltage and are functions of pulse voltage at higher voltages.[25,52] One investigator has found that reduction of tumor size varies directly with pulse length and the square of pulse voltage, indicating that the effects of electrochemotherapy may be a function of pulse energy.[51]

10.3.2.3   Clinical Studies

In a Phase I–II clinical trial including eight patients, head and neck squamous cell carcinomas were treated with four or eight square-wave pulses of 780 V in strength and 100 µs in duration across electrodes of 6 mm spacing.[26,57] Out of 40 treated nodules, 23 showed clinical complete response and 6 showed only partial response. Side effects were limited to short, painless muscle contractions at the time of the pulses. Electrochemotherapy has also been performed on patients with melanomas.[58]

10.3.3   ELECTROPORATION OF SKIN FOR TRANSDERMAL DRUG DELIVERY

Although transdermal drug delivery has the potential to be a noninvasive, user-friendly method of delivering drugs, its clinical use has found limited application due to the remarkable barrier properties of the outermost layer of the skin, the stratum corneum.[59,60] As a result, chemical, iontophoretic, ultrasonic, and other methods of enhancement have been studied as approaches to increase rates of transport. First reported in 1992,[61] application of low-duty-cycle, high-voltage pulses has been shown to have dramatic effects on skin properties, including large increases in transdermal transport of a variety of different compounds, including macromolecules.[30-33,53,62-74] These effects are believed to be caused by skin electroporation, involving transient structural changes in the intercellular lipid bilayers of the stratum corneum. Although both electroporation and iontophoresis involve electric fields, the two phenomena are fundamentally different. While iontophoresis acts primarily on the drug, involving skin structural changes as a secondary effect,[59,60] electroporation is expected to act directly on the skin, making transient changes in tissue permeability.

10.3.3.1 Increases in Molecular Transport across Skin

10.3.3.1.1 Transdermal Flux of Calcein

While electroporation of unilamellar, phospholipid cell membranes is well known, electroporation of the multilamellar, nonphospholipid bilayers found in the intercellular spaces of stratum corneum has only recently been investigated. To determine if electroporation of the stratum corneum occurs, human cadaver epidermis under physiological conditions was subjected to electric pulses which cause electroporation in other systems. Most work focused on the transdermal transport of calcein caused by low-voltage constant electric fields (iontophoresis) and high-voltage pulsed electric fields (hypothesized to involve electroporation). Because of the overall hydrophobic character and net negative charge of the stratum corneum, transdermal transport of negatively charged hydrophilic drugs is especially challenging. Therefore, calcein, a moderate-sized ($M_r = 623$ Da), highly polar ($z = -4$ net charge) molecule,[75] was selected as a model drug because its transport across skin is particularly difficult.

The effects of exposing human epidermis *in vitro* to exponential-decay electric field pulses (decay time constant, $\tau = 1$ ms) at a rate of 12 pulses/min is shown in Figure 10.6A as a function of voltage.[30] Fluxes before pulsing were below the detection limit (of order 10^{-4} mg/cm^{2}h, imposed by background fluorescence), while fluxes during pulsing were up to four orders of magnitude above this limit. Flux increased nonlinearly with increasing pulse voltage; that is, flux increased strongly with increasing voltage below approximately 100 V and increased weakly with increasing voltage at higher voltages.

Transdermal calcein transport due to electric field pulses of both forward polarity and alternating polarity is shown (Figure 10.6A).[30] Here, forward-polarity pulses correspond to the positive electrode in the receptor compartment and the negative electrode in the donor compartment. For this configuration, electric field pulses could both cause structural changes in the skin, possibly due to electroporation, as well as move calcein across the skin by electrophoresis through both previously existing and newly created transport pathways. In contrast, alternating-polarity pulses were applied such that the electrode polarity alternated with each pulse. Although each pulse was either completely positive or completely negative, the total time integral of voltage over all pulses was zero. Both forward- and alternating-polarity pulses resulted in significant increases in transdermal flux.

Theoretical analysis of skin electroporation has predicted that the multilamellar lipid bilayers of human stratum corneum could electroporate at voltages on the order of 100 V.[76,77] The resulting predictions of one model[77,78] are shown in Figure 10.6A. This model, which accounts for the geometric and physiochemical properties of the skin and the compounds being transported, was developed from first principles and

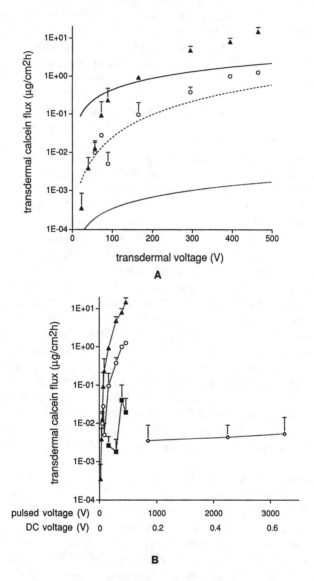

FIGURE 10.6

requires no fitted parameters. It has previously been shown[78] to predict passive and
low-voltage iontophoretic transport across skin. The lower, dotted curve represents
the prediction of the model for calcein transport during forward-polarity pulses
through unaltered skin; the prediction of the model is very poor. In contrast, the
upper, solid line represents the prediction for transport across skin containing transient pores, having characteristics consistent with what is known about single-bilayer
electroporation; the prediction is much better. Finally, the middle, dashed line

represents the prediction for transport during alternating-polarity pulses through porated skin, which is also in good agreement with the data. This analysis both shows that a theoretical basis exists for changes in skin structure and establishes that these changes are capable of explaining some of the characteristic effects of high-voltage pulsing.

Enhancement of transdermal transport at low voltage (e.g., <1 V) can generally be explained by electrophoresis and/or electro-osmosis without changes in skin structure.[79,80] Therefore, if protocols having the same electrophoretic and electro-osmotic driving force provide different degrees of enhancement, it suggests that changes in skin properties occurred. Fluxes caused by low-duty-cycle, high-voltage pulsing were therefore compared with fluxes caused by continuous low voltages which would provide the same total electrophoretic and electro-osmotic driving force. Transport enhancement by electrophoresis or electro-osmosis is proportional to the time integral of voltage.[81] Therefore, continuous application of 0.1 V should provide the same driving force as 500 V applied at a 1:5000 duty cycle (1-ms pulse applied once every 5 s). As seen in Figure 10.6B, application of continuous DC voltages caused fluxes three orders of magnitude smaller than pulsing under "equivalent" forward-polarity conditions. Moreover, while alternating-polarity pulses also dramatically increased transport, no enhancement resulted from equivalent low-voltage AC current which provided the same time-averaged driving force for transport (data not shown).[70] Finally, increases in transport of two orders of magnitude have been seen when the polarity is such that electrophoresis and electro-osmosis oppose transdermal transport (Figure 10.6B). These comparisons suggest that electrophoresis and/or electro-osmosis alone cannot explain the large flux increases observed during high-voltage pulsing, which indicates that changes in skin properties occurred.

One of the key features of electroporation seen in single-bilayer membranes is dramatically increased transport by a mechanism involving structural changes in the

---

FIGURE 10.6 Experimental data and theoretical predictions for the transdermal flux of calcein under different electrical conditions. (A) Calcein flux during forward-polarity (▲) and alternating-polarity (○) pulses (see text for definitions). Flux was increased by up to four orders of magnitude. Theoretical predictions are also shown for transport across unaltered skin during forward-polarity pulsing (dotted line), transport across skin containing electropores during forward-polarity pulsing (solid line), and transport across skin with electropores during alternating-polarity pulsing (dashed line). (B) Calcein flux during forward-polarity (▲), alternating-polarity (○), and reverse-polarity (■) pulsing and during DC iontophoresis (◊). The upper axis indicates pulsing voltage electrically "equivalent" to continuous DC voltages on the lower axis (see text). Dotted lines connecting the points in each data set are shown to aid the reader, but have no physical interpretation. For both graphs, fluxes represent average values during 1 h of electrical exposure. Either a continuous DC voltage or a series of intermittent (12 pulses/min) exponential-decay pulses ($\tau = 1$ to 1.3 ms) was applied to human epidermis *in vitro*. Standard deviation bars are shown. (Compiled from Prausnitz, M. R. et al., *Proc. Natl. Acad. Sci. U.S.A.*, 90, 10504, 1993, Prausnitz, M. R. et al., *J. Controlled Release*, 38, 205, 1996, and Edwards, D. A. et al., *J. Controlled Release*, 34, 211, 1995. With permission.)

membrane barrier.[1,3] Figure 10.6 suggests that this is seen in skin, too. A second feature of electroporation is that over a range of conditions, these changes are reversible.[1,3] This is also seen in skin. In experiments that identified long-lived changes in skin permeability, pulses at or below approximately 100 V were shown to cause no detectable long-lived changes in skin permeability, while higher voltage pulses appeared to cause lasting changes,[30] which did not go away, even after 18 to 24 h.

Experiments performed to assess the combined effects of electroporation and ultrasound (1 MHz, 1.4 W/cm^2, continuous application) on skin found a synergistic effect which increased transdermal flux two- to threefold and reduced transport lag time compared with electroporation alone.[65] Both ultrasound-induced lipid bilayer disordering and cavitation-related convection may have contributed to the increased effects of electroporation. Ultrasound also lowered the minimum voltage required for electroporation-induced flux increases by 13%,[65] possibly due to partial disordering of lipid bilayer structure by ultrasound.

Finally, limited work on electroporation *in vivo* has been performed on hairless rats,[30,53] assessed by measuring serum concentrations of calcein delivered transdermally. At voltages between 30 and 300 V, fluxes in excess of 10 μg/cm^{2}h were observed, which is at least two orders of magnitude greater than controls. *In vivo* fluxes did not increase with voltage, suggesting that a rate-limiting step other than transport across the stratum corneum existed, perhaps uptake of calcein from a skin depot into the bloodstream. No visible skin damage was observed after pulsing at voltages below 150 V; erythema and edema were evident at higher voltages. Long-term biochemical and pathological studies are needed.

10.3.3.1.2   Transport Number Analysis

Transport numbers represent the fraction of total current carried by a given ionic species, which can be regarded as the efficiency of electrophoretic transport of that species.[81,82] By calculating the transport number ($t_{calcein}$), or transport efficiency, associated with different electrical conditions, the pathways available to ion transport can be partially characterized. Here, $t_{calcein}$ is a measure of the efficiency with which calcein can be transported through pathways across skin relative to transport of small ions, such as sodium or chloride. Thus, transport numbers can give information about the effective average size of transport pathways.

During both iontophoresis and high-voltage pulsing, $t_{calcein}$ has been shown to increase with increasing current and voltage (Figure 10.7).[70] This means that the changes in skin properties caused by increased current or voltage increase transport of calcein more than small ions, perhaps due to creation of larger transport pathways. At the lowest voltages and currents, small ion transport was favored over calcein transport by a factor of 1000 ($t_{calcein} \approx 10^{-5}$, compared with the predicted maximum value, corresponding to pathways much larger than calcein, $t_{calcein, max} \approx 10^{-2}$)[70] (Figure 10.7). Under these conditions, transport pathways may have dimensions similar to that of calcein (Stokes–Einstein radius, $r_{calcein} = 0.6$ nm).[77] In this case, transport of small ions such as sodium or chloride (crystal ionic radius, $r_{Na^+} = 0.1$ nm and $r_{Cl^-} = 0.2$ nm)[83] would be less hindered, while calcein would experience considerable steric hindrance. Pathways that might show this selectivity could include

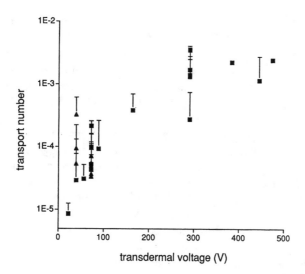

FIGURE 10.7 Transport number for calcein transport across human epidermis *in vitro* during exponential-decay pulses (■) and square-wave pulses (▲). For each point, pulses of a constant duration between 30 µs and 1 ms were applied for 1 h at a constant rate between 10^{-1} and 10^4 pulses/min. Transport number, which is a measure of the efficiency with which the electric field transported calcein, increased with increasing voltage. Standard deviation bars are shown. (From Prausnitz, M. R. et al., *J. Controlled Release,* 38, 205, 1996. With permission.)

transport between intercellular lipid bilayers of the stratum corneum ($r = 0.7$ nm)[84] or through intercellular junctions in the lining of shunt pathways. Another possibility is that many pathways exist that only allow small-ion transport, such as angstrom-size "leaks" in lipid bilayers created by random thermal motion,[85] along with a few much larger routes which readily permit passage of calcein, perhaps associated with appendages.

At the highest voltages and currents, where $t_{calcein}$ approached its predicted maximum value ($t_{calcein, max} \approx 10^{-2}$)[70] (Figure 10.7), larger pathways may exist, with dimensions much larger than calcein. In this case, small-ion transport would remain unhindered while calcein transport would become less hindered. This would increase $t_{calcein}$ by increasing calcein transport relative to small ions. However, with this data alone, the absolute size of these pathways or whether they were newly created or enlargements of preexisting pathways cannot be assessed.

Finally, $t_{calcein}$ has been shown to have no clear dependence on pulse length, rate, energy, waveform, or total charge transferred.[70] This is consistent with known mechanisms of single-bilayer electroporation, where pore characteristics are believed to be determined largely by voltage.[1,3]

10.3.3.1.3   Transdermal Flux of Other Compounds

While many skin electroporation studies have been performed with calcein as a model drug, electroporation-enhanced transport of a number of other molecules has also been reported. By using a protocol similar to that described for calcein, enhanced transport of three other moderate-sized, polar molecules across skin has been achieved by electroporation: Lucifer Yellow (M_r = 457 Da, z = −1 net charge),[30] sulforhodamine (M_r = 607 Da, z = −1 net charge),[33] and an erythrosin derivative (M_r = 1025 Da, z = −2 net charge).[30] By using a different protocol, involving fewer but longer and somewhat lower-voltage pulses, electroporation has been shown to increase transport of metoprolol (M_r = 267 Da, z = +1 net charge)[32,69] and fentanyl (M_r = 336 Da, z = +1 net charge).[86]

In studies of metoprolol flux across electroporated hairless rat skin *in vitro*,[32,69] the mechanism of transport was found to be diffusion through permeablized skin during the pulsing protocol. Collection of drug in reservoirs within the skin was also found to be significant. Transdermal transport was determined to increase directly with pulse length (above a threshold of 80 ms) and with the square of pulse voltage for a series of low-voltage (less than ~65 V across the skin), long-duration (τ > 80 ms) exponential-decay pulses. This may suggest that transport was a function of applied energy.[69] However, this dependence on energy did not apply when other protocols were used (e.g., square-wave or higher-voltage pulses).[32,69]

More recently, transport of macromolecules has been shown to be enhanced by electroporation. By using a protocol similar to that used in the calcein studies, oligo-nucleotides (M_r = 4.8 and 7 kDa)[64] and heparin (see discussion below)[71] were transported across skin *in vitro* at therapeutically useful rates. Moreover, using a protocol which applied a single initial electroporation pulse which was followed by iontophoresis, the transport of luteinizing hormone–releasing hormone (LHRH; M_r = 1182 Da, z = +1 net charge),[31] (arg^8)-vasopressin (M_r = 1084 Da, z = +2 net charge),[87] and neurotensin (M_r = 1693 Da, z = +1 net charge)[87] were also enhanced by electroporation.

LHRH flux is shown in Figure 10.8 as a function of current density of ionto-phoresis following a single exponential-decay electroporation pulse (300 to 400 V, τ = 5 to 9 ms) or iontophoresis alone.[31] The application of a single pulse caused changes in skin permeability such that flux during subsequent iontophoresis was an order of magnitude greater. Calculation of transport numbers from those data show a tenfold increase following electroporation,[31] indicating that the high-voltage pulse resulted in larger transdermal transport pathways.

Heparin is a macromolecule (M_r = 5 to 30 kDa) in widespread clinical use which is often administered by continuous infusion, due to the poor oral bioavailability of heparin, its short half-life, and the risk of bleeding complications.[88] Transdermal delivery of heparin would be a desirable alternative, if heparin could be transported across skin at therapeutic rates. Under passive conditions (no electric fields) trans-dermal heparin flux is negligible.[71] However, while applying short (τ = 1.9 ms), high voltage (150 to 350 V across skin) pulses to the skin at a rate of 12 pulses/min, rates of transdermal heparin transport were between 100 and 500 mg/cm^{2}h (Figure 10.9A). This level of transport is therapeutically relevant (see below). Moreover, heparin transported across the skin was biologically active (Figure 10.9A).

Constant current iontophoresis (0.1 to 1 mA/cm^2) also enhanced heparin trans-port, but to a much lesser extent (Figure 10.9A). The currents used during low-voltage iontophoresis were selected for two reasons. First, they bracketed the max-imum current density (~0.5 mA/cm^2) which patients tolerate during clinical ionto-phoresis.[89] Second, the time-averaged current passed during high-voltage pulsing

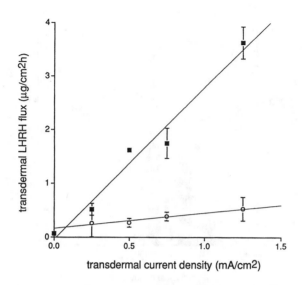

FIGURE 10.8 Transdermal transport of LHRH as a function of current density due to iontophoresis following a single electroporation pulse (■) and due to iontophoresis alone (○). This figure suggests that the application of a single electroporation pulse before iontophoresis can significantly increase the flux of LHRH relative to iontophoresis alone. Pre-iontophoresis pulses were exponential decay ($\tau = 5$ ms) and applied 1000 V across the electrodes. Linear regressions are shown. (From Bommannan, D. B. et al., *Pharm. Res.,* 11, 1809, 1994. With permission.)

was in the range of 0.1 to 1 mA/cm^2.[71] Therefore, both low- and high-voltage protocols had the same time-averaged current and therefore passed the same number of ionic charges across the skin, making comparisons of transport efficiency (i.e., transport number analysis) more direct.

Heparin transport numbers during high-voltage pulsing ($t_{heparin} = 0.054 \pm 0.006$) were calculated to be about an order of magnitude greater than during iontophoresis ($t_{heparin} = 0.007 \pm 0.002$) (Figure 10.9B) . These values indicate that approximately 5% of the current was carried by heparin during pulsing, compared with only 0.7% during iontophoresis.[71] This significant difference in transport numbers implies that heparin transport was significantly less hindered during high-voltage pulsing than during iontophoresis, perhaps because high-voltage pulses caused transient changes in skin microstructure by creating new and/or enlarged aqueous pathways for transport across the skin, and thereby increasing $t_{heparin}$. Low-voltage iontophoresis does not cause these changes in skin structure[59,60] and, therefore, has less effect on $t_{heparin}$. Nevertheless, all measured transport numbers were significantly less than the maximum value ($t_{heparin} = 1$),[71] indicating that although heparin transport was less hindered during high-voltage pulsing, in all cases transport was still significantly hindered. Unless transport pathways are extremely large (i.e., much larger than a heparin molecule), this is expected.[71]

The heparin fluxes reported during high-voltage pulsing (100 to 500 µg/cm^{2}h or 2 to 10 U/cm^{2}h) are therapeutically relevant. For example, administration from a

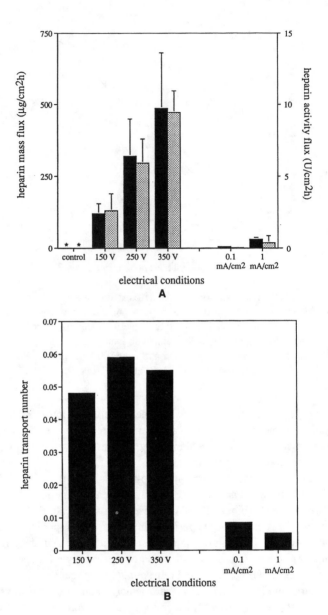

FIGURE 10.9

100-cm^2 patch would result in a heparin delivery rate of 10 to 50 mg/h or 200 to 1000 U/h, based on mass flux and activity flux measurements, respectively (Figure 10.9A). This is in the range sufficient for low-dose prophylaxis of thromboembolism (~500 U/h)[88] and full-dose anticoagulation therapy (700 to 2000 U/h).[88]

10.3.3.1.4   Rapid Temporal Control by Electroporation

To better understand the kinetics of transdermal transport by electroporation, a flow-through system has been designed which can give temporal resolution approaching 10 s.[90] By using this system, transdermal transport by electroporation of calcein and sulforhodamine across human epidermis was continuously measured (Figure 10.10).[33] For calcein, the flux reached a steady state within minutes and then decreased below background levels within seconds after pulsing stopped. In contrast, sulforhodamine flux increased continuously during pulsing and did not return to background levels after pulsing.[33]

At first, the curve for calcein flux may appear to contain a lot of noise. However, closer examination shows that the flux oscillated with a regular period of 1 peak/min.[62,67] This is the same rate at which pulses were applied, suggesting that these variations show the effects on transport of individual pulses. This is supported by results seen while pulsing at other rates, where oscillations in flux also occurred at the same rate as pulsing.[33,62,67] As a result of each pulse, the flux initially increased and then decayed as the effects of the pulse decreased. From this and other data, the steady-state lag time for calcein was determined to be the time it took to apply approximately 10 pulses (i.e., in Figure 10.10, where 1 pulse was applied each minute, the lag time was about 10 min), independent of voltage.[62] Moreover, the onset time for transport was the time it took to give 3 pulses, independent of voltage: in Figure 10.10, the first detectable transdermal transport was measured after 3 min.[62]

The pulse-dependent oscillation in calcein flux suggests that calcein was transported primarily during individual pulses.[90] The smooth curve for sulforhodamine flux indicates that sulforhodamine was continuously transported both during and between pulses. Mechanistically, this suggests that calcein transport occurs primarily by electrophoresis during pulses, and not by diffusion between pulses.[33,65] Given the moderate size of calcein ($M_r = 623$ Da) and its great charge ($z = -4$), this is reasonable. In contrast, sulforhodamine transport could occur largely by diffusion between pulses. Given its much weaker charge ($z = -1$), this is also reasonable.

Because the transport of calcein has been shown to be rapidly responsive to the electric field, electroporation protocols have been designed to achieve desired delivery profiles.[62] For example, continuous low-level delivery of a drug with intermittent

---

FIGURE 10.9   Flux and transport number of transdermal heparin transport during different electrical protocols. (A) Transdermal heparin flux determined by different assays. Heparin mass flux (■) was determined by radioactivity measurements, while biological activity flux (▨) was determined by the whole blood recalcification time assay.[103] In all cases, active heparin was transported across the skin. Standard deviation bars are shown. Asterisk indicates a flux below the detection limit (of order 1 μg/cm²h for radioactivity measurements and 0.1 U/cm²h for biological activity measurements). (B) Heparin transport number during different electrical protocols. During high-voltage pulsing, transport numbers were approximately 0.05, while during low-voltage iontophoresis they were about an order of magnitude smaller. The larger transport numbers seen during high-voltage pulsing suggest the creation of larger aqueous pathways by the electric field. (From Prausnitz, M. R. et al., *Bio/Technology*, 13, 1205, 1995. With permission.)

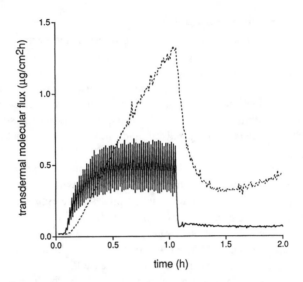

FIGURE 10.10 Simultaneous measurement of the transdermal flux of calcein (M_r = 623 Da, z = –4 net charge; solid line) and sulforhodamine (M_r = 607 Da, z = –1 net charge; dashed line) using a continuous flow-through apparatus. Calcein flux rapidly reached a quasi-steady state and oscillated at a frequency equal to the pulse rate. In contrast, sulforhodamine flux neither oscillated nor reached a steady state. These differences can be explained by calcein transport primarily by electrophoresis during pulses and sulforhodamine transport primarily by diffusion between pulses (see text). Exponential-decay pulses (decay time constant, τ = 1.1 ms) causing a peak transdermal voltage of 200 V were applied to human epidermis *in vitro* at a rate of 1 pulse/min for 1 h. (From Pliquett, U. and Weaver, J. C., *Bioelectrochem. Bioenerget.*, 39, 1, 1996. With permission.)

boli may be a desirable delivery schedule for some drugs. To achieve this type of delivery, iontophoresis was applied to supply baseline delivery, while electroporation pulses provided rapid boli (Figure 10.11A). A more complex delivery profile is shown in Figure 10.11B. In these figures, changes in delivery rates were achieved by changing pulse voltage. However, changes in pulse rate can also achieve similar results.[33,67] Finally, by using an initial series of pulses applied more rapidly to "prime the pump," followed by less rapid pulsing to provide the desired steady-state flux, steady state was achieved within approximately 1 min.[62]

10.3.3.2 Changes in Skin Electrical Properties

Measuring changes in skin electrical properties can give insight into the mechanism of changes in transport properties and the nature of transport pathways. During the application of high-voltage pulses to human epidermis *in vitro*, skin dynamic resistance has been determined as a function of voltage (Figure 10.12).[33,66] Below 40 V, millisecond-long pulses had little effect on resistance. However, at higher voltages the skin dynamic resistance dropped two to three orders of magnitude within microseconds during each pulse. This corresponds to extensive creation or enlargement of pathways for ionic current across the skin.

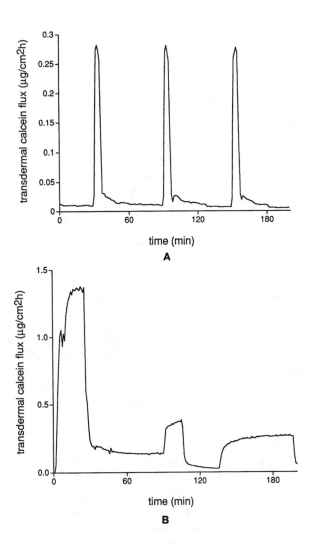

FIGURE 10.11 Complex delivery profiles using transdermal delivery by electroporation. (A) Continuous low-level delivery with intermittent boluses. Low-level delivery corresponded to continuous DC iontophoresis at 14 mA/cm². Boli corresponded to pulsing at 115 V and 12 pulses/min for 5 min, each separated by 55 min of iontophoresis. (B) A complex delivery schedule achieved by changing pulse voltage. Pulse rate was held constant at 1 pulse/min, while pulse voltage was changed in the following sequence: 270 V for 30 min, 115 V for 60 min, 165 V for 15 min, 0 V for 30 min, 135 V for 60 min, 0 V for 5 min. Exponential-decay pulses (decay time constant, $\tau = 1$ ms) were applied to human epidermis *in vitro*. (From Prausnitz, M. R. et al., *Pharm. Res.*, 11, 1834, 1994. With permission.)

Measurements of human skin resistivity made milliseconds after application of a single pulse show recovery from about 100 Ω-cm² to on the order of 10,000 Ω-cm².[33,66,74] Then, within 1 s further recovery occurs, usually bringing skin resistance to within 50% of its prepulse value. This recovery has been observed to occur independent

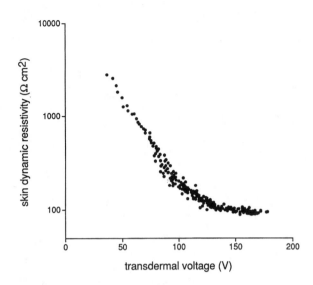

FIGURE 10.12   Skin dynamic resistivity during the application of a high-voltage pulse shown as a function of peak transdermal voltage. On a time scale of microseconds or less, skin dynamic resistivity dropped by two to three orders of magnitude (prepulse skin resistivity was on the order of 100,000 kΩ cm^2). Resistivity changes were generally reversible for pulses between 40 and 100 V. Pulses greater than 100 V were only partially reversible, while pulses less than 40 V caused insignificant changes in skin resistivity. Dynamic resistance was determined 20 μs after the onset of an exponential-decay pulse ($\tau = 1$ ms) applied to human epidermis *in vitro*. (From Pliquett, U. et al., *Biochim. Biophys. Acta*, 1239, 111, 1995. With permission.)

of voltage after single pulses.[66] After 1 s, over a time scale of minutes, skin resistance can recover further, exhibiting either complete or partial recovery. At the highest voltages, recovery after ~1 s occurs to a much less extent. The time scales and degrees of both onset and recovery are characteristic of known electrical properties of single-bilayer electroporation.[1,3]

These dramatic but largely reversible effects of electroporation can be compared with the effects of a well-accepted medical procedure: a needle stick. Puncturing and removing from the skin a small needle (28 gauge) caused skin resistance drops which were not reversible and were at least as great as those caused by skin electroporation at the highest voltages.[74] This suggests that although electroporation is not fully reversible under all conditions, the irreversible changes it causes may be less damaging than the effects of a small needle.

When multiple pulses are applied to the skin, resistance continues to drop with each successive pulse until 15 to 30 pulses have been applied, after which additional pulses do not decrease resistance further.[33,66] As the number of pulses and the rate at which they are applied are increased, skin dynamic resistance during pulsing and the degree of recovery after pulsing both decrease. When many (e.g., 100) multiple pulses are applied at high voltage, skin resistance may return to only 10% of its prepulse value, indicating significant irreversibility.

Measurements made immediately after high-voltage pulsing have also shown up to sixfold increases in skin capacitance which later recover to prepulse values.[33,66,74] Capacitance has been found to increase with the square of voltage,[66,74] suggesting an energy-dependent mechanism. Increased capacitance may indicate changes in skin lipids[91] since skin capacitance is generally attributed to stratum corneum lipid bilayers.[92,93] In contrast, low-voltage electric fields have been shown to cause no or much smaller changes in skin capacitance.[79,93,94]

The combination of calcein transport and skin electrical property measurements allows estimation of what fraction of the skin is available to ion transport and over what characteristic times transport pathways become accessible. By measuring skin resistance and assuming that ion transport pathways are filled with saline, the area fraction of skin made up of these pathways, F_{ion}, has been estimated.[70] After minutes to hours of conventional iontophoresis (up to a few volts), human skin resistivity can drop to between 1000 and 10,000 Ω-cm^2).[79,80,95,96] This corresponds to ion transport pathways occupying an estimated 0.01 to 0.001% of skin surface area ($F_{ion} \approx 10^{-5}$ to 10^{-4}).[70] This is the same area occupied by hair follicles and sweat ducts in human skin,[97] consistent with these shunt routes being the sites of transport during iontophoresis, as shown previously.[98-100]

Making the same calculation for high-voltage pulses, during which skin resistance drops to approximately 100 Ω-cm^2,[33,66,70,74] indicates that about 0.1% of skin surface area becomes available to ion transport ($F_{ion} \approx 10^{-3}$).[33,70] Electroporation of single bilayers is also believed to cause poration of up to 0.1% of membrane area.[101,102] These estimates suggest that 10 to 100 times more skin area is available for ion transport during high-voltage pulsing than conventional iontophoresis. This may correspond to a shift from iontophoretic transport largely through shunt routes to transport predominantly through electropores within the bulk of stratum corneum.

Differences between pathways available to small ions and those available to calcein can also be considered. Because F_{ion} gives the fraction of skin area containing ion pathways and the ratio $t_{calcein}/t_{calcein, max}$ gives the fraction of ion pathways available to calcein transport, then the fraction of skin area available to calcein transport ($F_{calcein}$) can be estimated as the product of these two quantities.[70] By using this relationship, $F_{calcein}$ was estimated to range from 10^{-6} to 10^{-3} during high-voltage pulsing and from 10^{-8} to 10^{-4} during iontophoresis.[33,70]

Finally, the timescale over which these transport pathways become accessible has been estimated. Changes in skin resistance due to conventional iontophoretic exposures generally occur over a characteristic time of at least minutes.[79,80,95,96] In contrast, ion transport pathways created by high-voltage pulses become accessible at least eight orders of magnitude more quickly, within a characteristic time of microseconds.[33,66,70,74] Electroporation of single bilayers is also known to occur on a timescale of microseconds or faster.[1,3] Given that high-voltage pulsing causes a one to two order of magnitude greater reduction of resistance that occurs at least eight orders of magnitude more quickly than is typical for iontophoresis, it seems unlikely that the mechanistic bases for changes associated with the two protocols are the same.

10.3.3.3   Microscopic Imaging of Transdermal Transport

Fluorescence microscopy has been used to understand more fully the nature, size, and location of transport pathways in skin exposed to high-voltage pulses. In these studies, human skin was exposed to fluorescent probes (calcein and/or sulforho-damine) and electrical protocols *in vitro* using either (1) a side-by-side permeation chamber, from which skin was later removed and examined by scanning confocal fluorescence microscopy[73] or (2) a chamber placed on a conventional fluorescence microscope stage, allowing real-time microscopic evaluation.[68] After iontophoresis at currents up to 1 mA/cm^2, calcein was seen to be heterogeneously transported into the stratum corneum, as revealed by occasional large areas (measuring on the order of 100 μm across) which were more brightly labeled than the surrounding tissue.[73] While fluorescence generally appeared to be intercellular, a signal was sometimes seen to originate from within the interior of keratinocytes. The typical hexagonal outlines of cells were always evident within the brightly labeled regions, suggesting that no gross morphological changes had occurred. Cross-sectional images showed that calcein was present throughout the stratum corneum.[73]

High-voltage pulses applied to the skin resulted in bright regions of similar dimensions to those found after iontophoresis (Figure 10.13A).[68,73] Both intercellular and intracellular fluorescence was observed. Outlines of cellular structures were also evident.[73] Additional experiments showed that the sites of skin fluorescence corresponded to both sites of molecular transport across (as opposed to just into) the skin and paths of ionic current.[68] Moreover, these sites did not correspond to sweat ducts or hair follicles. Transport regions covered between 0.02 and 8% of skin area. Closer examination[68] by digital image analysis revealed that each fluorescent region contained several subpeaks of fluorescence, suggesting additional microstructure within these transport regions.

FIGURE 10.13   Micrographs of human stratum corneum showing fluorescence of calcein transported by high-voltage pulsing *in vitro*. Sites of fluorescence can be interpreted as sites of transdermal calcein transport. (A) Localized transport regions can be seen, having dimensions of 50 to 100 μm. Ten exponential-decay pulses ($\tau = 1$ ms) causing a peak transdermal voltage of 157 V were applied to human epidermis at a rate of 2 pulses/min. This signal-averaged image was collected immediately after the application of pulses using a fluorescence microscope with a digital video-imaging system. Scale bar equals 200 μm. (From Pliquett, U. F. et al., *Biophys. Chem.*, 58, 185, 1996. With permission). (B) A close-up view of a localized transport region, showing a brightly fluorescent area with a nonfluorescent interior, or fluorescent "ring." Exponential-decay pulses (decay time constant, $\tau = 1.1$ ms) causing a peak transdermal voltage of 300 V were applied to human epidermis *in vitro* at a rate of 12 pulses/min for 1 h. Skin samples were flash-frozen and later imaged using scanning confocal fluorescence microscopy. Scale bar equals 50 μm. (From Prausnitz, M. R. et al., *J. Pharm. Sci.*, 85, 1363, 1996. With permission.)

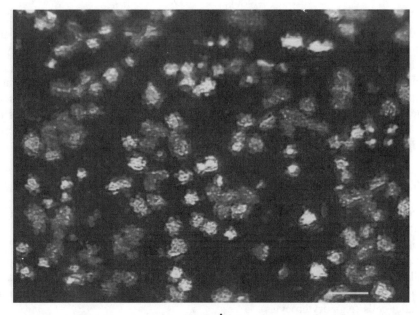

A

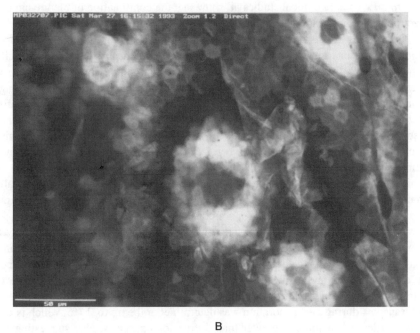

B

FIGURE 10.13

Unlike iontophoresis or pulsing at lower voltages, pulsing at higher voltage (e.g., 300 V across the skin) led to the appearance of bright regions containing dark interiors, i.e., fluorescent "rings" (Figure 10.13B).[73] These rings were never observed in iontophoretic or lower-voltage pulsed samples and were always found in samples pulsed at 300 V. A series of additional experiments[73] involving lipophilic stains and fluorescent nanospheres suggested that while the fluorescent outer rings represent sites of transport which retained calcein, the dark ring interiors represent sites of transport which did not retain calcein at the time of imaging, possibly because of long-lasting local structural changes of nanometer dimensions.

10.4 CONCLUSIONS

Electroporation involves the creation of transient aqueous pathways in lipid bilayer membranes by the application of a short electric field pulse and has been observed in isolated cells and in tissues, including tumors and the skin stratum corneum. For drug delivery, electroporation has been shown to be capable of loading red blood cells with a model drug that can later be released *in vivo*. Moreover, electroporation can selectively permeabilize larger cells (e.g., leukocytes) among a population of smaller cells (e.g., erythrocytes).

In applications that enhance cancer chemotherapy with bleomycin, electroporation of tumors results in increased drug uptake due to membrane permeabilization. *In vitro*, *in vivo*, and clinical studies all show that the combination of bleomycin and electroporation kills tumor cells and often results in complete regression.

Different from isolated cells and cells part of a tissue (e.g., tumors), electroporation of skin for transdermal drug delivery involves permeabilization of the multilamellar, intercellular lipid bilayers in the stratum corneum. Flux increases up to four orders of magnitude have been observed with human skin *in vitro* for a range of hydrophilic molecules up to thousands of daltons in molecular mass (e.g., heparin, oligonucleotides). Sites of transport have been observed to be heterogeneously distributed across the skin. Electroporation-mediated transport is rapidly responsive to changes in electrical conditions, where (1) skin transport properties change over a time scale of microseconds or faster and (2) steady-state transdermal flux can be achieved on a time scale of minutes. Skin electroporation has also been theoretically characterized, indicating that changes in transport due to electroporation of lipid bilayers within the stratum corneum are consistent with experimental results.

Comparison of transdermal transport during low-voltage, constant electric fields (iontophoresis) and high-voltage pulsed electric fields (electroporation) indicated that the transport enhancement seen during electroporation could not be explained by electrophoresis and/or electro-osmosis alone, but suggested the occurrence of skin structural changes. Moreover, the estimated area fraction of skin available to ion transport during electroporation was determined to be up to 0.1%, which is one to two orders of magnitude greater than during iontophoresis, also suggesting the creation (or enlargement) of transport pathways. While a variety of mechanisms could be proposed to explain these results, transient changes in skin structure created by a mechanism related to electroporation is offered as the most-promising hypothesis.

ACKNOWLEDGMENTS

Thanks to D. B. Bommannan, U. Pliquett, and R. Vanbever for help with manuscript preparation and insightful discussions. This work was supported in part by The Whitaker Foundation for Biomedical Engineering.

REFERENCES

1. Neumann, E., Sowers, A. E., and Jordan, C. A., Eds., *Electroporation and Electrofusion in Cell Biology*, Plenum Press, New York, 1989.
2. Tsong, T. Y., Electroporation of cell membranes, *Biophys. J.*, 60, 297–306, 1991.
3. Chang, D. C., Chassy, B. M., Saunders, J. A., Sowers, A. E., and Chang, D. C., Eds., *Guide to Electroporation and Electrofusion*, Academic Press, New York, 1992.
4. Orlowski, S. and Mir, L. M., Cell electropermeabilization: a new tool for biochemical and pharmacological studies, *Biochim. Biophys. Acta*, 1154, 51–63, 1993.
5. Weaver, J. C., Electroporation: a general phenomenon for manipulating cells and tissues, *J. Cell. Biochem.*, 51, 426–435, 1993.
6. Chernomordik, L. V., Sukharev, S. I., Abidor, I. G., and Chizmadzhev, Y. A., The study of the BLM reversible electrical breakdown mechanism in the presence of UO_2^{2-}, *Bioelectrochem. Bioenerget.*, 9, 149–155, 1982.
7. Dimitrov, D. S. and Sowers, A. E., Membrane electroporation — fast molecular exchange by electroosmosis, *Biochim. Biophys. Acta*, 1022, 381–392, 1990.
8. Prausnitz, M. R., Lau, B. S., Milano, C. D., Conner, S., Langer, R., and Weaver, J. C., A quantitative study of electroporation showing a plateau in net molecular transport, *Biophys. J.*, 65, 414–422, 1993.
9. Dev, S. B. and Hofmann, G. A., Electrochemotherapy — a novel method of cancer treatment, *Cancer Treat. Rev.,* 20, 105–115, 1994.
10. Benz, R. F., Beckers, F., and Zimmermann, U., Reversible electrical breakdown of lipid bilayer membranes: a charge-pulse relaxation study, *J. Membrane Biol.*, 48, 181–204, 1979.
11. Serpersu, E. H., Kinosita, K., and Tsong, T. Y., Reversible and irreversible modification of erythrocyte membrane permeability by electric field, *Biochim. Biophys. Acta*, 812, 770–785, 1985.
12. Hibino, M., Shigemori, M., Itoh, H., Nagayama, K., and Kinosita, K., Jr., Membrane conductance of an electroporated cell analyzed by submicrosecond imaging of transmembrane potential, *Biophys. J.*, 59, 209–220, 1991.
13. Klenchin, V. A., Sukharev, S. I., Serov, S. M., Chernomordik, L. V., and Chizmadzhev, Y. A., Electrically induced DNA uptake by cells is a fast process involving DNA electrophoresis, *Biophys. J.*, 60, 804–811, 1991.
14. Prausnitz, M. R., Corbett, J. D., Gimm, J. A., Golan, D. E., Langer, R., and Weaver, J. C., Millisecond measurement of transport during and after an electroporation pulse, *Biophys. J.*, 68, 1864–1870, 1995.
15. Maurel, P., Gualandris-Parisot, L., Teissié, J., and Duprat, A.-M., *Exp. Cell. Res.*, 184, 207–218, 1989.
16. Kwee, S., Nielsen, H. V., and Celis, J. E., Electropermeabilization of human cultured cells grown in monolayers, *Bioelectrochem. Bioenerget.*, 23, 65–80, 1990.
17. Pu, H. and Young, A. P., *Gene*, 89, 259–263, 1990.
18. Yaseen, M. A., Pedley, K. C., and Howell, S. L., *Biochem. J.*, 206, 81–87, 1982.

19. Persaud, S. J., Jones, P. M., and Howell, S. L., *Biochem. J.*, 258, 669–675, 1989.
20. Dekeyser, R. A., Claes, B., De Rycke, R. M. U., Habets, M. E., Van Montagu, M. C., and Caplan, A. B., Transient gene expression in intact and organized tissues, *Plant Cell*, 2, 591–602, 1990.
21. D'Hulluin, K., Bonne, E., Bossut, M., De Beuckeleer, M., and Leemans, J., Transgenic maize plants by tissue electroporation, *Plant Cell*, 4, 1495–1505, 1992.
22. Bhatt, D. L., Gaylor, D. C., and Lee, R. C., Rhabdomyolysis due to pulsed electric fields, *Plast. Reconstr. Surg.*, July, 1–11, 1990.
23. Okino, M. and Mohri, H., Effects of a high voltage electrical impulse and an anti-cancer drug on in vivo growing tumors, *Jpn. J. Cancer Res.*, 78, 1319–1321, 1987.
24. Kanesada, H., Anticancer effect of high voltage pulses combined with concentration dependent anticancer drugs on Lewis lung carcinoma, in vivo, *Jpn. J. Soc. Cancer. Ther.*, 25, 2640–2648, 1990.
25. Mir, L. M., Orlowski, S., Belehradek, J., and Paoletti, C., Electrochemotherapy potentiation of antitumor effect of bleomycin by local electric pulses, *Eur. J. Cancer*, 27, 68–72, 1991.
26. Belehradek, M., Domenge, C., Luboinski, B., Orlowski, S., Belehradek, J., and Mir, L. M., Electrochemotherapy, a new antitumor treatment, *Cancer*, 72, 3694–3700, 1993.
27. Salford, L. G., Persson, B. R. R., Brun, A., Ceberg, C. P., Kongstad, P. C., and Mir, L. M., A new brain tumour therapy combining bleomycin with in vivo electropermeabilization, *Biochem. Biophys. Res. Commun.*, 194, 938–943, 1993.
28. Titomirov, A. V., Sukharev, S., and Kistanova, E., In vivo electroporation and stable transformation of skin cells of newborn mice by plasmid DNA, *Biochim. Biophys. Acta*, 1088, 131–134, 1991.
29. Powell, K. T., Morgenthaler, A. W., and Weaver, J. C., Tissue electroporation: observation of reversible electrical breakdown in viable frog skin, *Biophys. J.*, 56, 1163–1171, 1989.
30. Prausnitz, M. R., Bose, V. G., Langer, R., and Weaver, J. C., Electroporation of mammalian skin: a mechanism to enhance transdermal drug delivery, *Proc. Natl. Acad. Sci. U.S.A.*, 90, 10504–10508, 1993.
31. Bommannan, D., Tamada, J., Leung, L., and Potts, R. O., Effect of electroporation on transdermal iontophoretic delivery of luteinizing hormone releasing hormone (LHRH) in vitro, *Pharm. Res.*, 11, 1809–1814, 1994.
32. Vanbever, R., Lecouturier, N., and Préat, V., Transdermal delivery of metoprolol by electroporation, *Pharm. Res.*, 11, 1657–1662, 1994.
33. Pliquett, U. and Weaver, J. C., Electroporation of human skin: simultaneous measurement of changes in the transport of two fluorescent molecules and in the passive electrical properties, *Bioelectrochem. Bioenerget.*, 39, 1–12, 1996.
34. Abidor, I. G., Arakelyan, V. B., Chernomordik, L. V., Chizmadzhev, Y. A., Pastushenko, V. F., and Tarasevich, M. R., Electric breakdown of bilayer membranes: I. The main experimental facts and their qualitative discussion, *Bioelectrochem. Bioenerget.*, 6, 37–52, 1979.
35. Barnett, A. and Weaver, J. C., A unified, quantitative theory of reversible electrical breakdown and rupture, *Bioelectrochem. Bioenerget.*, 25, 163–182, 1991.
36. Weaver, J. C. and Barnett, A., Progress toward a theoretical model for electroporation mechanism: membrane electrical behavior and molecular transport, in *Guide to Electroporation and Electrofusion*, D. C. Chang, B. M. Chassy, J. A. Saunders, and A. E. Sowers, Eds., Academic Press, New York, 1992, 91–118.

37. Weaver, J. C. and Chizmadzhev, Y. A., Theory of electroporation: a review, *Bioelectrochem. Bioenerget.*, 41, 135–160, 1996.
38. Chang, D. C. and Reese, T. S., Changes in membrane structure induced by electroporation as revealed by rapid-freezing electron microscopy, *Biophys. J.*, 58, 1–12, 1990.
39. Langer, R., New methods of drug delivery, *Science*, 249, 1527–1533, 1990.
40. Müller, R. H., *Colloidal Carriers for Controlled Drug Delivery and Targeting*, Wissenschaftliche Verlagsgesellschaft, Stuttgart, 1991.
41. Kydonieus, A., Ed., *Treatise on Controlled Drug Delivery*, Marcel Dekker, New York, 1992.
42. Zimmermann, U., Riekmann, F., and Pilwat, G., Enzyme loading of electrically homogeneous human red blood cell ghosts prepared by dielectric breakdown, *Biochim. Biophys. Acta*, 436, 460–474, 1976.
43. Kinosita, K., Jr. and Tsong, T. Y., Survival of sucrose-loaded erythrocytes in the circulation, *Nature*, 272, 258–260, 1978.
44. Sixou, S. and Teissie, J., Specific electropermeabilization of leucocytes in a blood sample and application to large volumes of cells, *Biochim. Biophys. Acta*, 1028, 154–160, 1990.
45. Jain, R. K., Physiological resistance to the treatment of solid tumors, in *Drug Resistance in Oncology*, B. A. Teicher, Ed., Marcel Dekker, New York, 1993, 87–105.
46. Orlowski, S., Belehradek, J., Paoletti, C., and Mir, L. M., Transient electropermeabilization of cells in culture. Increase of the cytotoxicity of anticancer drugs, *Biochem. Pharmacol.*, 37, 4727–4733, 1988.
47. Poddevin, B., Orlowski, S., Belehradek, J., and Mir, L. M., Very high cytotoxicity of bleomycin introduced into the cytosol of cells in culture, *Biochem Pharmacol*, 42, Suppl., S67-S75, 1991.
48. Okino, M. and Esato, K., The effects of a single high voltage electrical stimulation with an anticancer drug on in vivo growing malignant tumors, *Jpn. J. Surg.*, 20, 197–204, 1990.
49. Belehradek, J., Orlowski, S., Poddevin, B., Paoletti, C., and Mir, L. M., Electrochemotherapy of spontaneous mammary tumors in mice, *Eur. J. Cancer*, 27, 73–76, 1991.
50. Okino, M., Tomie, H., Kanesada, H., Marumoto, M., Morita, N., Esato, K., and Suzuki, H., Induction of tumor specific selective toxicity in electrical impulse chemotherapy — analysis of dose-response curve, *Oncologia*, 24, 71–79, 1991.
51. Okino, M., Tomie, H., Kanesada, H., Marumoto, M., Esato, K., and Suzuki, H., Optimal electric conditions in electrical impulse chemotherapy, *Jpn. J. Cancer Res.*, 83, 1095–1101, 1992.
52. Belehradek, J., Orlowski, S., Ramirez, L. H., Pron, G., Poddevin, B., and Mir, L. M., Electropermeabilization of cells in tissues assessed by the qualitative and quantitative electroloading of bleomycin, *Biochim. Biophys. Acta*, 1190, 155–163, 1994.
53. Prausnitz, M. R., Seddick, D. S., Kon, A. A., Bose, V. G., Frankenburg, S., Klaus, S. N., Langer, R., and Weaver, J. C., Methods for in vivo tissue electroporation using surface electrodes, *Drug Delivery*, 1, 125–131, 1993.
54. Mir, L. M., Orlowski, S., Poddevin, B., and Belehradek, J., Electrochemotherapy tumor treatment is improved by interleukin-2 stimulation of the host's defenses, *Eur. Cytokine Netw.*, 3, 331–334, 1992.
55. Mir, L. M., Roth, C., Orlowski, S., Belehradek, J., Fradelizi, F., Paoletti, C., and Kourilsky, P., Potentiation of the antitumoral effect of electrochemotherapy by an immunotherapy with allogenic cells producing interleukin 2, *C. R. Acad. Sci.* (Paris), 314, 539–544, 1992.

56. Mir, L. M., Roth, C., Orlowski, S., Quintin-Colonna, F., Fradelizi, D., Belehradek, J., and Kourilsky, P., Systemic antitumor effects of electrochemotherapy combined with histoincompatible cells secreting interleukin-2, *J. Immunother. Emphasis Tumor Immunol.*, 17, 30–38, 1995.

57. Mir, L. M., Belehradek, M., Domenge, C., Orlowski, S., Poddevin, B., Belehradek, J., Schwaab, G., Luboinski, B., and Paoletti, C., Electrochemotherapy, a novel antitumor treatment: first clinical trial, *C. R. Acad. Sci.* (Paris), Sér III 313, 613–618, 1991.

58. Heller, R., Treatment of cutaneous nodules using electrochemotherapy, *J. Fla. Med. Assoc.*, 82, 147–150, 1995.

59. Bronaugh, R. L. and Maibach, H. I., Eds., *Percutaneous Absorption, Mechanisms — Methodology — Drug Delivery*, Marcel Dekker, New York, 1989.

60. Hadgraft, J. and Guy, R. H., Eds., *Transdermal Drug Delivery: Developmental Issues and Research Initiatives*, Vol. 35, Marcel Dekker, New York, 1989.

61. Prausnitz, M. R., Bose, V. G., Langer, R., and Weaver, J. C., Transdermal drug delivery by electroporation, *Proc. Int. Symp. control. Rel. Bioact. Mater.*, 19, 232–233, 1992.

62. Prausnitz, M. R., Pliquett, U., Langer, R., and Weaver, J. C., Rapid temporal control of transdermal drug delivery by electroporation, *Pharm. Res.*, 11, 1834–1837, 1994.

63. Prausnitz, M. R., Bose, V. G., Langer, R., and Weaver, J. C., Electroporation, in *Percutaneous Penetration Enhancers,* E. W. Smith and H. I. Maibach, Eds., CRC Press, Boca Raton, FL, 1995, 393–405.

64. Zewert, T. E., Pliquett, U. F., Langer, R., and Weaver, J. C., Transdermal transport of DNA antisense oligonucleotides by electroporation, *Biochem. Biophys. Res. Commun.*, 212, 286–292, 1995.

65. Kost, J., Pliquett, U., Mitragotri, S., Yamamoto, A., Langer, R., and Weaver, J., Enhanced transdermal drug delivery: synergistic effect of electroporation and ultrasound, *Pharm. Res.*, 13, 633–638, 1996.

66. Pliquett, U., Langer, R., and Weaver, J. C., Changes in the passive electrical properties of human stratum corneum due to electroporation, *Biochim. Biophys. Acta*, 1239, 111–121, 1995.

67. Pliquett, U. and Weaver, J. C., Transport of a charged molecule across the human epidermis due to electroporation, *J. Controlled Release*, 38, 1–10, 1996.

68. Pliquett, U., Zewart, T. E., Chen, T., Langer, R., and Weaver, J. C., Imaging of fluorescent molecule and small ion transport through human stratum corneum during high voltage pulsing: localized transport regions are involved., *Biophys. Chem.*, 58, 185–204, 1996.

69. Vanbever, R. and Preat, V., Factors affecting transdermal delivery of metoprolol by electroporation, *Bioelectrochem. Bioenerget.*, 38, 223–228, 1995.

70. Prausnitz, M. R., Lee, C. S., Liu, C. H., Pang, J. C., Singh, T.-P., Langer, R., and Weaver, J. C., Transdermal transport efficiency during skin electroporation and iontophoresis, *J. Controlled Release*, 38, 205–217, 1996.

71. Prausnitz, M. R., Edelman, E. R., Gimm, J. A., Langer, R., and Weaver, J. C., Transdermal delivery of heparin by skin electroporation, *Bio/Technology*, 13, 1205–1209, 1995.

72. Prausnitz, M. R., Do high-voltage pulses cause changes in skin structure? *J. Controlled Release*, 40, 321–326, 1996.

73. Prausnitz, M. R., Gimm, J. A., Guy, R. H., Langer, R., Weaver, J. C., and Cullander, C., Imaging of transport pathways across human stratum corneum during high-voltage and low-voltage electrical exposures, *J. Pharm. Sci.*, 85, 1363–1370, 1996.

74. Bose, V. G., *Electrical Characterization of Electroporation of Human Stratum Corneum*, Ph.D. Thesis, Massachusetts Institute of Technology, Cambridge, MA, 1994.

75. Furry, J. W., *Preparation Properties and Applications of Calcein in a Highly Pure Form*, Ph.D. Thesis, Iowa State University, Ames, IA, 1985.

76. Chizmadzhev, Y. A., Zarnytsin, V. G., Weaver, J. C., and Potts, R. O., Mechanism of electroinduced ionic species transport through a multilamellar lipid system, *Biophys. J.*, 68, 749–765, 1995.

77. Edwards, D. A., Prausnitz, M. R., Langer, R., and Weaver, J. C., Analysis of enhanced transdermal transport by skin electroporation, *J. Controlled Release*, 34, 211–221, 1995.

78. Edwards, D. A. and Langer, R., A linear theory of transdermal transport phenomena, *J. Pharm. Sci.*, 83, 1315–1334, 1994.

79. Dinh, S. M., Luo, C.-W., and Berner, B., Upper and lower limits of human skin electrical resistance in iontophoresis, *AIChE J.*, 39, 2011–2018, 1993.

80. Inada, H., Ghanem, A.-H., and Higuchi, W. I., Studies on the effects of applied voltage and duration on human epidermal membrane alteration/recovery and the resultant effects upon iontophoresis, *Pharm. Res.*, 11, 687–697, 1994.

81. Bockris, J. O. and Reddy, A. K. N., *Modern Electrochemistry*, Vol. 1, Plenum Press, New York, 1970.

82. Phipps, J. B. and Gyory, J. R., Transdermal ion migration, *Adv. Drug Delivery Rev.*, 9, 137–176, 1992.

83. Weast, R. C., Ed., *CRC Handbook of Chemistry and Physics*, CRC Press, Boca Raton, FL, 1985.

84. Bouwstra, J. A., de Vries, M. A., Gooris, G. S., Bras, W., Brussee, J., and Ponec, M., Thermodynamic and structural aspects of the skin barrier, *J. Controlled Release*, 15, 209–220, 1991.

85. Weaver, J. C., Powell, K. T., Mintzer, R. A., Sloan, S. R., and Ling, H., The diffusive permeability of bilayer membranes: the contribution of transient aqueous pores, *Bioelectrochem. Bioenerget.*, 12, 405–412, 1984.

86. Vanbever, R., Le Boulengé, E., and Préat, V., Transdermal delivery of fentanyl by electroporation. I. Influence of electrical factors, *Pharm. Res.*, 13, 559–565, 1996.

87. Tamada, J., Sharifi, J., Bommannan, D. B., Leung, L., Azimi, N., Abraham, W., and Potts, R., Effect of electroporation on the iontophoretic delivery of peptides in vitro, *Pharm. Res.*, 10, S-257, 1993.

88. Majerus, P. W., Broze, G. I., Miletech, J. P., and Tollefsen, D. M., Anticoagulant, thrombolytic, and antiplatelet drugs, in *The Pharmacological Basis of Therapeutics*, 8th ed., A. G. Gilman, T. W. Rall, A. S. Nies, and P. Taylor, Eds., Pergamon Press, New York, 1990, 1311–1334.

89. Ledger, P. W., Skin biological issues in electrically enhanced transdermal delivery, *Adv. Drug Delivery Rev.*, 9, 289–307, 1992.

90. Pliquett, U., Prausnitz, M. R., Chizmadzhev, Y. A., and Weaver, J. C., Measurement of rapid release kinetics for drug delivery, *Pharm. Res.*, 12, 549–555, 1995 (Errata in *Pharm. Res.*, 12, 1244, 1995).

91. Potts, R. O., Guy, R. H., and Francoeur, M. L., Routes of ionic permeability through mammalian skin, *Solid State Ionics*, 53–56, 165–169, 1992.

92. DeNuzzio, J. D. and Berner, B., Electrochemical and iontophoretic studies of human skin, *J. Controlled Release*, 11, 105–112, 1990.

93. Oh, S. Y., Leung, L., Bommannan, D., Guy, R. H., and Potts, R. O., Effect of current, ionic strength and temperature on the electrical properties of skin, *J. Controlled Release*, 27, 115–125, 1993.

94. Yamamoto, T. and Yamamoto, Y., Non-linear electrical properties of skin in the low frequency range, *Med. Biol. Eng. Comput.*, 19, 302–310, 1981.

95. Kasting, G. B., Theoretical models for iontophoretic delivery, *Adv. Drug Delivery Rev.*, 9, 177–199, 1992.

96. Prausnitz, M. R., The effects of electric current applied to the skin: a review for transdermal drug delivery, *Adv. Drug Delivery Rev.*, 18, 395–425, 1996.

97. Champion, R. H., Burton, J. L., and Ebling, F. J. G., Eds., *Textbook of Dermatology*, Blackwell Scientific, London, 1992.

98. Cullander, C. and Guy, R. H., Sites of iontophoretic current flow into the skin: identification and characterization with the vibrating probe electrode, *J. Invest. Dermatol.*, 97, 55–64, 1991.

99. Cullander, C., What are the pathways of iontophoretic current flow through mammalian skin? *Adv. Drug Delivery Rev.*, 9, 119–135, 1992.

100. Scott, E. R., Laplaza, A. I., White, H. S., and Phipps, J. B., Transport of ionic species in skin: contribution of pores to the overall skin conductance, *Pharm. Res.*, 10, 1699–1709, 1993.

101. Rosemberg, Y. and Korenstein, R., Electroporation of the photosynthetic membrane: a study by intrinsic and external optical probes, *Biophys. J.*, 58, 823–832, 1990.

102. Freeman, S. A., Wang, M. A., and Weaver, J. C., Theory of electroporation of planar membranes: predictions of the aqueous area, change in capacitance and pore-pore separation, *Biophys. J.*, 67, 42–56, 1994.

103. Freed, L. E., Vunjak-Norakovic, G. V., Drinker, P. A., and Langer, R., Bioreactor based on suspended particles of immobilized enzyme, *Ann. Biomed. Eng.*, 21, 57–65, 1993.

11 Phonophoresis

Joseph Kost

CONTENTS

11.1 INTRODUCTION

In spite of major research and development efforts in transdermal systems and the many advantages of the transdermal route, impermeability of the human skin is still a major problem that limits the usefulness of the transdermal approach. It is well accepted that the stratum corneum is the major rate-limiting barrier to molecular diffusion through the mammalian epidermis.[1,2] Due to the fact that most drugs do not permeate the skin in therapeutic amounts, chemical and physical approaches have been examined to lower the stratum corneum barrier properties and enhance transdermal permeation.[3,4]

Although chemical approaches using molecules, such as dimethyl sulfoxide (DMSO), 1-dodecylazacycloheptan-2-one (azone) surfactants, solvents, and binary polar and apolar systems, have been shown to provide enhancement, many have not been widely accepted either because of suspected pharmacological activity or unresolved questions about safety.[5] In addition to the chemical approach, several physical approaches for skin penetration enhancement have been evaluated, such as stripping of the stratum corneum, thermal energy, iontophoresis, electroporation, and ultrasound.

Phonophoresis or sonophoresis is defined as the movement of drugs through living intact skin and into soft tissue under the influence of an ultrasonic perturbation.[6-10] This chapter attempts to present phonophoresis, experimental variables, and possible mechanisms of action, and the most representative experimental and clinical studies.

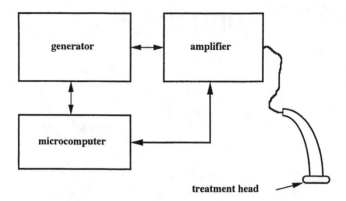

FIGURE 11.1   General schematic of ultrasonic equipment.

11.2   ELEMENTARY PHYSICS OF ULTRASONIC WAVES

Ultrasound is defined as any sound which is of a frequency beyond 20 KHz. Most modern ultrasound equipment is based on the piezoelectric effect. When pressure is applied to crystals (quartz), and some polycrystalline materials such as lead-zircon-ate-titanium (PZT) and barium titanate, electric charges develop on the outer surface of the material. The piezoelectric effect, which is reversible, was discovered in 1880 by the Curie brothers.[12,13] Thus, rapidly alternating potential when applied across opposite faces of a piezoelectric crystal will induce corresponding alternating, dimensional changes and thereby convert electrical into vibrational (sound) energy.

There are three distinctly different biomedical applications of ultrasound that can be identified in terms of their frequency ranges and applications:[14]

1. High-frequency or diagnostic ultrasound (2 to 10 MHz).
2. Medium-frequency or therapeutic ultrasound (0.7 to 3 MHz).
3. Low-frequency or power ultrasound (5 to 100 KHz).

The therapeutic ultrasound most frequently applied for transdermal drug delivery enhancement consists of a high-frequency generator which is connected to a piezo-electric crystal (the treatment head) (Figure 11.1). The resonant frequency of the crystal is partly determined by the thickness of the piezoelectric material, and consequently the frequency of the ultrasound is so determined as well.

11.2.1   PROPERTIES OF THE ULTRASOUND BEAM

The ultrasound beam has two distinctive areas: the near field (Fresnel zone) and the distant field (Fraunholer zone). The near field is characterized by interference phe-nomena in the ultrasound beam, which may lead to marked variations in intensity; these are expressed as the beam nonuniformity ratio (BNR). The distant field is characterized by the near absence of interference phenomena, so that the sound beam is uniform and the intensity gradually decreases with increasing distance. The length of the near field depends on the diameter of the treatment head and the wavelength. With the common treatment heads for therapeutic applications, the near field is about 10 cm long for a 5-cm^2 head and 1 cm long for a 1-cm^2 head at 1 MHz. At 3 MHz the near field is three times as long. Because the depth effect of ultrasound is limited, the therapeutic effects occur mainly in the near field.[14]

11.2.2 THE NATURE OF THE ULTRASOUND WAVE

The ultrasound wave is of a longitudinal nature; i.e., the direction of propagation is the same as the direction of oscillation.[14,15] The longitudinal sound waves cause compression and expansion of the medium at a distance of half a wavelength, leading to pressure variations in the medium. The wavelength of ultrasound is expressed by the relationship:

$$\lambda * f = C$$

where λ = wavelength
  f = frequency
  C = speed of propagation

In soft tissue and in water a wavelength of 1 MHz is approximately 1.5 mm, and in bony tissue it is about 3 mm. The medium is compressed and expanded at the same frequency as that of the ultrasound. At 1 MHz the resultant pressure changes are fairly large. For instance, at an intensity of 1 W/cm^2 the pressure variation is about 1.7 bar. At a wavelength of 1.5 mm, this implies a pressure gradient of 3.4 bar over a distance of 0.75 mm as the high and low pressures are half a wavelength apart.[14]

11.2.3 THE MASS DENSITY AND ACOUSTIC IMPEDANCE

The mass density of the medium (ρ) and the specific acoustic impedance (Z) determine the resistance of the media to sound waves. The mass density also partly determines the speed of the propagation (C). The higher the mass density, the higher the speed of propagation. The specific acoustic impedance, which is a material parameter, depends on the mass density and the speed of propagation $Z = \rho * C$. The specific acoustic impedance for skin, bone, and air are $1.6 * 10^6$, $6.3 * 10^6$, and 400 kg/m^2 s, respectively.[14]

11.2.4 ABSORPTION AND PENETRATION OF ULTRASOUND

As ultrasound energy penetrates into the body tissues, biological effects can be expected to occur only if the energy is absorbed by the tissues. The absorption coefficient (a) is used as a measure of the absorption in various tissues. For ultrasound consisting of longitudinal waves with perpendicular incidence on homogeneous tissues, the following formula applies:

$$I(x) = I_0 * e^{-ax}$$

where $I(x)$ = intensity at depth x

I_0 = intensity at the surface

a = absorption coefficient

A different value relating to absorption is the half-value depth ($D_{1/2}$), defined as the distance in the direction of the sound beam in which the intensity in a certain medium decreases by half. For skin the $D_{1/2}$ is 11.1 mm at 1 MHz and 4 mm at 3 MHz. In air $D_{1/2}$ is 2.5 mm at 1 MHz and 0.8 mm at 3 MHz.

To transfer the ultrasound energy to the body, it is necessary to use a contact medium because of the complete reflection of the ultrasound by air. The many types of contact media currently available for ultrasound transmission can be broadly classified as follows: oils, water oil emulsions, aqueous gels, and ointments.

11.3   CLINICAL STUDIES

Over the past 40 years numerous clinical reports have been published concerning phonophoresis. The technique involves placing the topical preparation on the skin over the area to be treated and massaging the area with an ultrasound probe. Some of the earliest studies done with phonophoresis involve hydrocortisone. Fellinger and Schmid[18] reported successful treatment of polyarthritis of the digital joints of the hand using hydrocortisone ointment with phonophoresis. Newman et al.[19] and Coodley[20] showed improved results of hydrocortisone injection combined with ultrasound "massage" compared with simple hydrocortisone injection for a bursitis treatment.

In addition to joint diseases and bursitis, phonophoresis has been tested for its ability to aid penetration in a variety of drug–ultrasound combinations, mainly for localized conditions. The major medications used include the anti-inflammatories, e.g., cortisol, dexamethasone, salicylates, and local anesthetics.[21] Cameroy[22] reported success using Carbocaine phonophoresis before closed reduction of Colles' fractures. Griffin et al.[23] treated 102 patients with diagnoses of elbow epicondylitis, bicipital tendonitis, shoulder osteoarthritis, shoulder bursitis, and knee osteoarthritis with hydrocortisone and ultrasound. Their results rated 68% of patients receiving drug in conjunction with ultrasound as "improved" demonstrating a pain-free normal functional range of motion, while only 28% of patients receiving placebo with ultrasound were rated as "improved." Similar effects were presented by Moll[24] who published a double-blind study with three groups of patients receiving lidocaine/decadron with ultrasound, or a placebo with ultrasound, or a placebo with ultrasound at zero intensity. Percentage improvement for the three groups were 88.1, 56.0, and 23.1%, respectively.

McElnay et al.[25] evaluated the influence of ultrasound on the percutaneous absorption of lignocaine from a cream base. Mean data indicated that there was a slightly faster onset time for local anesthesia when ultrasound was administered as compared with control values (no ultrasound). However, the differences were not statistically significant. In further studies performed by the authors[26] on percutaneous absorption of fluocinolone, ultrasound treatment led to enhanced percutaneous absorption.

Benson et al.[27] reported on the influence of ultrasound on the percutaneous absorption of lignocaine and prilocaine from Emla cream. The local anesthetic cream formulation Emla was chosen because it requires a relatively long contact time with the skin before the application site becomes anesthetized (60 min). The authors evaluated three frequencies (0.75, 1.5, and 3 MHz) at a continuous intensity of 1.5 W/cm^2 or frequencies of 1.5 or 3.0 MHz, 1:1 pulsed output, at an intensity of 1.0 W/cm^2. The 1.5-MHz (1:1 pulsed output) and 3.0-MHz (continuous output) ultrasound appeared to be the most effective frequencies in improving the rate of percutaneous absorption, while the 1.5-MHz and 3-MHz (1:1 pulsed output) ultrasound treatments were the most effective frequencies in improving the extent of drug absorption. Benson et al.[28,29] demonstrated that ultrasound is also capable of enhancing the percutaneous absorption of methyl and ethyl nicotinate. For the lipophilic hexyl nicotinates, no effect of ultrasound on its percutaneous absorption could be detected. The pharmacodynamic parameter of vasodilation caused by nicotinates was used to monitor percutaneous absorption. Recently, McEnlay et al.[30] evaluated the skin penetration enhancement effect of phonophoresis on methyl nicotinate in ten healthy volunteers in a double-blind, placebo-controlled, crossover clinical trial. Each treatment consisted of the application of ultrasound massage (3.0 MHz, 1.0 W/cm^2 continuous output) or placebo (0 MHz) for 5 min to the forearm, followed by a standardized application of methyl nicotinate at intervals of 15 s, 1 min, and 2 min ultrasound massage. Ultrasound treatment applied prior to methyl nicotinate led to enhanced percutaneous absorption of the drug. The authors suggest that the ultrasound affects the skin structure by disordering the structured lipids in the stratum corneum.

Similar experiments were performed by Hofman and Moll[31] who studied the percutaneous absorption of benzyl nicotinate. For recording the reddening of the skin a reflection photometry was employed. Ultrasonic treatment of the skin at levels lower than 1 W/cm^2 reduced the lag time as a function of ultrasound power. Repetition of the ultrasonic treatment confirmed the reversibility of the changes in skin permeability.

Kleinkort and Wood[32] compared phonophoretic effects of a 1% cortisol mixture to that of a 10% mixture. Although an improvement of approximately 80% of the patients receiving 1% cortisol was demonstrated, the group treated with the 10% mixture showed improvement in 95.7% of the patients and treatment of 16 patients with subdeltoid bursitis showed 100% improvement. In all groups, the 10% compound was more effective. The transmission characteristics of a number of topical proprietary preparations containing drugs suitable for use with ultrasound have been investigated by Benson and McElnay;[33] gel formulations were found to be the most suitable coupling agents.

Williams[34] developed an electrical sensory perception threshold technique for use with human volunteers in order to evaluate the effect of phonophoresis on three commonly available topical anesthetic preparations. Low intensities (0.25 W/cm^2) of 1.1-MHz ultrasound had no detectable effects upon the rate of penetration of any of the three anesthetic preparations through human skin under conditions where temperature increased had been minimized.

11.4 NONHUMAN *IN VIVO* STUDIES

Studies on phonophoresis of anti-inflammatories and local anesthetics were also performed on animals.[35-40] Kremkau[41] studied the effect of ultrasound and chemotherapeutic drugs in mouse leukemia. The treatment was applied *in vitro* with cells in suspension. The cells were inoculated into host mice and survival was monitored. The studies suggested the usefulness of ultrasound in chemotherapy, as the ultrasound localized the anticancer drugs to the desired area, increasing their effectiveness without increasing systemic toxicity.

Tachibana and Tachibana[42] applied ultrasound to deliver insulin through the skin of hairless mice partially immersed in an aqueous solution of insulin (20 U/mL). Two energy ranges, 3000 to 5000 Pa and 5000 to 8000 Pa, at a frequency of 48 kHz applied for 5 min were evaluated. The blood glucose concentration was measured before and after exposure to insulin and ultrasonic vibration. The blood glucose decreased to $34 \pm 11.9\%$ of control values in 120 min, while when exposed to the higher ultrasonic energy the glucose values fell to $22.4 \pm 3.9\%$ of the controls. The glucose concentrations remained low for the length of the experiment (240 min). Tachibana and Tachibana[43] also applied ultrasound to deliver lidocaine through the skin. Ultrasound exposure (5 min, 48 kHz, 0.17 W/cm^2) to the legs of hairless mice, immersed in a beaker containing 2% aqueous lidocaine, rapidly induced an anesthetic effect. Immersion in lidocaine without ultrasound or ultrasound in water without lidocaine showed no evidence of analgesia after treatment.

11.5 ULTRASOUND FOR TRANSDERMAL DELIVERY SYSTEMS

In the last decade, with the development of transdermal delivery as an important means of systemic drug administration, researchers investigated the possible application of ultrasound into transdermal delivery systems. Kost et al.[44-46] studied in rats and guinea pigs the effect of therapeutic ultrasound (1 MHz) on skin permeability of D-mannitol, a highly polar sugar alcohol, of inulin, a high-molecular-weight polysaccharide and of physostigmine, a lipophilic anticholinesterase drug. Ultrasound nearly completely eliminated the lag time usually associated with transdermal delivery of drugs; 3 to 5 min of ultrasound irradiation (1.5 W/cm^2 continuous wave or 3 W/cm^2 pulsed wave) increased the transdermal permeation of inulin and mannitol in rats by 5 to 20-fold within 1 to 2 h following ultrasound application (Figure 11.2). Ultrasound treatment also significantly increased the inhibition of cholinesterase during the first hour after application in both physostigmine-treated rats and guinea pigs.

Miyazaki et al.[47] performed similar studies evaluating the effect of ultrasound (1 MHz) on indomethacin permeation in rats. Pronounced effect of ultrasound on transdermal absorption for all three ranges of intensities (0.25, 0.5, and 0.75 W/cm^2) was observed.

Bommannan et al.[48,49] conducted *in vivo* experiments on hairless guinea pigs to test the ultrasound frequency effect on transdermal enhancement, postulating that

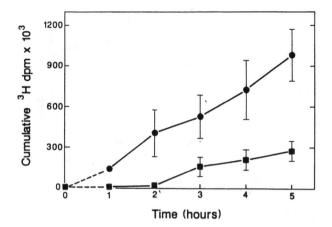

FIGURE 11.2 Cumulative radioactive secretion in rats after topical application of 20 μL of saturated solution of ᴅ-mannitol containing 20 μCi ᴅ-(3H)mannitol. (●) Ultrasound-treated rats *n* - 4. (1.5 W/cm² continuous wave for 3 min). (■) Control rats, no ultrasound, *n* = 12. (From Levy, D. et al., *J. Clin. Invest.*, 83, 2074, 1989. With permission.)

high-frequency ultrasound would improve the efficacy of ultrasound enhancement. The authors conclude:

1. Transdermal drug delivery of salicylic acid is significantly increased by ultrasound application for 5 or 20 min, when compared with passive diffusion.
2. The lag time associated with passive diffusion through the skin is significantly reduced.
3. Higher-frequency ultrasound can result in higher enhancement levels.

In contradiction to Bommannan and co-workers, Mitragotri et al.[50] presented a study where low-frequency ultrasound (20 kHz) was shown to increase the permeability of human skin to many drugs, including high-molecular weight proteins, such as insulin, interferon γ, and erythropoeitin, by several orders of magnitude. The authors also evaluated the sonophoretic enhancement of the low-frequency ultrasound on transdermal insulin transport *in vivo*, presenting ultrasound intensity-dependent decrease in the blood glucose concentration of hairless rats exposed to insulin and low-frequency ultrasound (Figure 11.3).

11.6 MECHANISM

A possible mechanism of improved percutaneous absorption by ultrasound suggested by several groups[29,47,51,52] is that ultrasound may interact with the structured lipids located in the intercellular channels of the stratum corneum. This is similar to the postulated effects of some chemical transdermal enhancers which act by disordering lipids.[53] The ultrasound energy may act to facilitate diffusion through lipid domains.

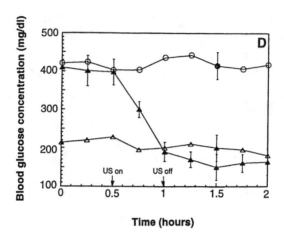

Time (hours)

FIGURE 11.3 Time variation of blood glucose concentration of diabetic hairless rats upon a 30-min insulin–ultrasound treatment (ultrasound, 20 kHz, 225 mW/cm^2, 100-ms pulses applied every second was turned on at 0.5 h and turned off at 1 h). Diabetic rats (○), normal rats(△), diabetic rats with insulin–ultrasound treatment(▲). (From Mitragotri, S. et al., *Science,* 269, 850, 1995. With permission.)

Various pathways of drug penetration have been associated with both stratum corneum proteins and lipids. The existence of corneocytes embedded in a lipid domain consisting of alternately hydrophilic and lipophilic layers suggested two major pathways for permeation across skin: one transcellular, the other via the tortuous but continuous path of intercellular lipids. Kost et al.[54] found that ultrasound enhanced the permeability through both the lipophilic and hydrophilic routes, suggesting that the effect of ultrasound on the lipoidal configuration is not the only contribution of ultrasound to the enhanced transdermal permeability. DSC and FTIR studies suggested that there were no irreversible morphological changes in the stratum corneum due to the ultrasound exposure.

Levy et al.[46] also performed *in vitro* studies to gain insight into the mechanism of ultrasonically enhanced transdermal delivery. The authors consider three factors that might contribute to the ultrasound-enhanced permeability: mixing, cavitation, and temperature. To examine whether ultrasound might affect a boundary layer in the neighborhood of the skin and therefore cause higher permeabilities, experiments were performed *in vitro* under controlled mixing rates. The temperature of the skin exposed to ultrasound was monitored. Cavitation effects were evaluated in *in vitro* permeability experiments in degassed buffer, where cavitation was minimized. The authors concluded that the small increase in surface skin temperature observed after ultrasound application (1 to 2°C) is not likely to cause dramatic changes in skin permeability. The ultrasound-enhancing phenomenon was mainly attributed to mixing and cavitation effects.

Mortimer et al.[55] showed that ultrasound exposure led to an increase in the rate of oxygen diffusion through frog skin. The authors found that the oxygen permeability increase is dependent upon the ultrasound average intensity, but does not depend on the peak acoustic pressure. Based on this finding, they conclude that it is not likely that cavitation is the dominant mode of action since cavitation mechanisms are a function of acoustic pressure rather than average intensity. In addition, transient cavitation was not observed through the measurement of OH radicals.[56] Since diffusion increased with increasing average intensity, the most likely mechanism proposed by the authors is acoustic streaming (quartz wind) leading to stirring action in the vicinity of the membrane, affecting the boundary layer (reducing the concentration gradient in the immediate neighborhood of the membrane).

Tachibana and Tachibana[42] postulated that the energy of ultrasonic vibration–enhanced transdermal permeability through the transfollicular and transepidermal routes. The microscopic bubbles (cavitation) produced at the surface of the skin by ultrasonic vibration might generate a rapid liquid flow when they implode, thereby increasing skin permeability.

Recently, Simonin[57] also suggested the sweat ducts as the main hydrophilic molecule passway affected by sonophoresis. Simonin, based on the calculations of the intercellular channels (0.01 to 0.1 μm) and intermingled filaments dense structure of the intracellular region, concludes that there is not enough space to allow for transient cavitation in the inter- or intracellular routes; cavitation, therefore, is unlikely to disrupt the orderly structure of the stratum corneum. In contrast, bubbles generated by ultrasound cavitation of the sweat duct lumen having a nominal diameter of about 5 μm can be formed and grow, possibly attaining their resonant size. Thereby, a vigorous mixing may be formed by microstreaming and bubble collapse, resulting in enhanced transport.

Bommannan et al.[49] examined the effects of ultrasound on the transdermal permeation of an electron-dense tracer, lanthanum nitrate. The results demonstrate that exposure of the skin to ultrasound can induce considerable and rapid tracer transport through an intercellular route. Prolonged exposure of the skin to high-frequency ultrasound (20 in, 16 MHz), however, resulted in structural alterations of epidermal morphology.

In a recent publication Mitragotri et al.[52] evaluated the role played by various ultrasound-related phenomena, including cavitation, thermal effects, generation of convective velocities, and mechanical effects. The authors' experimental findings suggest that among all the ultrasound-related phenomena evaluated, cavitation plays the dominant role in sonophoresis using therapeutic ultrasound (frequency, 1 to 3 MHz, intensity 0 to 2 W/cm^2). Confocal microscopy results indicate that cavitations occurs in the keratinocytes of the stratum corneum upon ultrasound exposure. The authors hypothesize that oscillations of the cavitation bubbles induce disorder in the stratum corneum lipid bilayers, thereby enhancing transdermal transport. The theoretical model developed to describe the effect of ultrasound on transdermal transport predicts that sonophoretic enhancement depends most directly on the passive permeant diffusion coefficient and not on the permeant diffusion coefficient through the skin.

Although it is difficult to be certain whether or not the data obtained in the *in vitro* experiments with synthetic polymeric membranes are extendable to the *in vivo* situation with skin, it is likely that, since both involve diffusion through membranes, those factors which ultrasound affects *in vitro* with synthetic polymeric membranes also play a role *in vivo*.

Three possible mechanisms were proposed by Howkins[58] by which ultrasound could influence the rate of permeability through a polymeric membrane: (1) the direct heating of the membrane; (2) the sinusoidal pressure variations across the membrane producing some rectifications of flow and thus small net dissolved permeant; (3) the reduction of the effect of weak forces between the membranes and the molecules diffusing through it. However, the results indicated that none of the suggested mechanisms is feasible and the authors concluded that the major effect was due to stirring of fluid layers next to the membranes.

Fogler and Lund[59] proposed that the enhancement of mass transport by ultrasound was due to ultrasonically induced convective transport created by acoustic streaming in addition to diffusional transport. Acoustic streaming is a secondary flow which produces time-independent vortices when an acoustic wave is passed through the medium.[60] The formation of these vortices or cells inside ducts, tubes, and pores can increase the rate of mass transfer through these enclosures. Between adjacent cells, molecular diffusion is the only means of mass transport; however, within each cell, transport is primarily by convection. A differential mass transport equation was coupled with the second-order time-independent streaming equation in a rectangular membrane duct which was solved by finite-difference techniques. The acoustic streaming strongly modifies the concentration field which would be present when only diffusional mass transfer takes place. An analytical solution of the proposed model showed that with the application of ultrasound an increase of up to 150% above the normal diffusive transport could be obtained.

Kost et al.[61] proposed enhanced protein blotting based on application of ultrasound; 3 min of ultrasound exposure (1 MHz, 2.5 W/cm^2) was sufficient for a very clear transfer of proteins from a polyacrylamide gel to nitrocellulose or nylon 66 membrane. The authors also propose that the enhancement of mass transport by ultrasound in the polymeric synthetic membranes is due to ultrasonically induced convective transport created by acoustic streaming.

Lenart and Auslander[62] found that ultrasound enhances the diffusion of electrolytes through cellophane membranes. They proposed the mechanism to be diminution of the hydration sphere surrounding the electrolytes, thus increasing the electrolyte mobility and diffusion coefficient. The authors also proposed a local temperature effect due to the implosion of cavitation bubbles to be a possible mechanism.

Julian and Zentner[63] systematically investigated the effect of ultrasound on solute permeability through polymer films. In these studies, the known parameters of permeation were controlled. Diffusivity of benzoic acid in polydimethylsiloxane films and hydrocortisone in cellulose films was increased 14% and 23%, respectively with 23-W ultrasound. The increase in permeability was unique to the ultrasonic pertubation and was not attributed to disruption of stagnant aqueous diffusion layers, increased membrane/solution temperature, or irreversible changes in membrane integrity. Recently, the authors[64] suggested the ultrasonically enhanced diffusion to be a result of a decrease of the activation energy necessary to overcome the potential energy barriers within the solution–membrane interfaces.

Kost et al.[65,66] suggested the feasibility of ultrasonic controlled implantable polymeric delivery systems in which the release rates of substances can be repeatedly modulated at will from a position external to the delivery system. Both bioerodible and nonerodible polymers were found to be responsive to the ultrasound; enhanced polymer erosion and drug release were noted when the delivery systems were exposed to ultrasound. The authors[67,68] proposed cavitation and acoustic streaming to be the mechanism of the enhanced polymer degradation and drug release.

11.7 CONCLUSIONS

The possibility for using ultrasound to mediate and enhance transdermal delivery of diverse substances of wide-ranging molecular size and chemical composition has appealing therapeutic and commercial possibilities. As most of the reported results applied ready-made ultrasonic units which were not designed for this specific application, there is no doubt that specifically designed units will enable higher transdermal permeability mediation which will lead to the preparation of transdermal delivery patches linked to miniature power sources that can be externally adjusted for a wide range of clinical applications. The recent results on the enhancing effect of low-frequency ultrasound on protein permeability suggest the possible future application of this approach for needless injections of proteins such as insulin, which is of very large interest. Such efforts at developing miniature and relatively inexpensive power sources will also be important for patient use and convenience.

In spite of the large number of studies that has been published recently on the effect of ultrasound on skin and synthetic membranes *in vivo* and *in vitro*, the mechanism of the enhancing phenomenon is still not well understood and characterized. The main factors contributing to this phenomenon include mixing, temperature, cavitation, acoustic streaming, and membrane morphological changes. As these are complex phenomena involving several parameters that are difficult to separate, carefully designed studies accompanied by theoretical approaches are essential in order to have the knowledge needed to design and optimize ultrasonically driven transdermal drug delivery systems.

REFERENCES

1. Scheuplein, R. J., Blank, I. H., Permeability of the skin. *Physiol. Rev.* 1971; 51:702–747.
2. Bartek, M., LaBudde, J., Maibach, H., Skin permeability in vitro: comparison in rat, rabbit, pig and man. *J. Invest. Dermatol.* 1972; 58:114.
3. Rolf, D., Chemical and physical methods of enhancing transdermal drug delivery. *Pharm. Technol.* 1988; 130–139.
4. Hadgraft, J., Guy, R. H., *Transdermal Drug Delivery.* Marcel Dekker, New York, 1989.
5. Walters, K. A., Penetration enhancers and their use in transdermal therapeutic systems. In Hadgraft, J., Guy, H. G., Eds., *Transdermal Drug Delivery, Developmental Issues and Research Initiatives.* Marcel Dekker, New York, 1989; 197–246.
6. Skauen, D. M., Zentner, G. M. Phonophoresis. *Int. J. Pharm.* 1984; 20:235–245.
7. Quillen, W. S., Phonophoresis: a review of the literature and technique. *Athl. Training* 1980; 15:109–110.

8. Tyle, P., Agrawala, P., Drug delivery by phonophoresis. *Pharm. Res.* 1989; 6:355–361.
9. Kost, J., Langer, R., Ultrasound-mediated transdermal drug delivery, in *Topical Drug Bioavailability, Bioequivalence, and Penetration,* Shah, V. P. and Maibach, H. I., Eds., Plenum Press, New York, 1993.
10. Sun, Y., Liu, I.-L., Transdermal drug delivery by phonophoresis: basic mechanisms, and techniques of application. *Drug Pharm. Sci.,* 1994; 62:303–321.
11. Camel, E., Ultrasound, in *Percutaneous Penetration Enhancers,* Smith, E. W. and Maibach, H. I., Eds., CRC Press, Boca Raton, FL, 1995, Chap. 15.2.
12. Curie, J., Curie, P., *Compt. Rend.* 1881; 93:1137.
13. Curie, J., Curie, P., *Compt. Rend.* 1880; 91:294.
14. Hoogland, R., *Ultrasound Therapy.* Enraf Nonius, Delft, Holland, 1986.
15. Sislick, K. S., *Ultrasound Its Chemical, Physical and Biological Effects.* VCH Publishers, Weinheim, 1988.
16. Mason, T. J., *Chemistry with Ultrasound.* Elsevier Applied Science, London, 1990.
17. Wells, P. N. T., *Biomedical Ultrasonics.* Academic Press, New York, 1977.
18. Fellinger, K., Schmid, J., Klinik and Therapies des chronischen Gelenkhreumatismus. *Maudrich* 1954; 549–552.
19. Newman, M. K., Kill, M., Frompton, G., The Effect of Ultrasound alone and combined with hydrocortisone injections by needle or hypospray, *Am. J. Phys. Med.* 1958; 37:206–209.
20. Coodley, G. L., Bursitis and post-traumatic lesions. *Am. Pract.* 1960; 11:181–187.
21. Antich, T. J., Phonophoresis: the principles of the ultrasonic driving force and efficacy in treatment of common orthopaedic diagnoses. *J. Ortho. Sports Phys. Ther.* 1982; 4:99–102.
22. Cameroy, B. M., Ultrasound enhanced local anasthesia. *Am. J. Orthoped.* 1966; 8:47.
23. Griffin, J. E., Echternach, J. L., Price, R. E., Touchstone, J. C., Patients treated with ultrasonic drive hydrocortisone and with ultrasound alone. *Phys. Ther.* 1967; 47:594–601.
24. Moll, M. A., A new approach to pain. *U.S. Armed Forces Med. Serv. Dig.* 1979; 30:8–11.
25. McElnay, J. C., Matthews, M. P., Harland, R., McCafferty, D. F., The effect of ultrasound on the percutaneous absorption of lignocaine. *Br. J. Clin. Pharmacol.* 1985; 20:421–424.
26. McElnay, J. C., Kennedy, T. A., Harland, R., The influence of ultrasound on the percutaneous absorption of fluocinolone acetonide. *Int. J. Pharm.* 1987; 40:105–110.
27. Benson, H. A. E., McElnay, J. C., Harland, R., Phonophoresis of lignocaine and prilocaine from Emla cream. *Int. J. Pharm.* 1988; 44:65–69.
28. Benson, H. A. E., McElnay, J. C., McCallion, O., Harland, R., Murphy, T. M., Hadgraft, J., Influence of ultrasound on the percutaneous absorption of a range of nicotinate esters. *J. Pharm. Pharmacol.* 1989; 40:40.
29. Benson, H. A. E., McElnay, J. C., Harland, R., Hadgraft, J., Influence of ultrasound on the percutaneous absorption of nicotinate esters. *Pharm. Res.* 1991; 8:204–209.
30. McEnlay, J. C., Benson, H. A. E., Harland, R., and Hadgraft, J., Phonophoresis of methyl nicotinate: a preliminary study to elucidate the mechanism. *Pharm. Res.* 1993; 4:1726–1731.
31. Hofman, D., Moll, F., The effect of ultrasound on in vitro liberation and in vivo penetration of benzyl nicotinate, *J. Controlled Release* 1993; 27: 185–192.
32. Kleinkort, J. A., Wood, F., Phonophoresis with 1 percent versus 10 percent hydrocortisone. *Phys. Ther.* 1975; 55:1320–1324.

33. Benson, H. A. E., McElnay, J. C., Transmission of ultrasound energy through topical pharmaceutical products. *Physiotherapy* 1988; 74:587–589.

34. Williams, A. R., Phonophoresis: an in vivo evaluation using three topical anaesthetic preparations. *Ultrasonics* 1990; 28:137–141.

35. Tsitlanazde, V. G., Morphohistochemical changes during experimental arthritis in rabbits caused by hydrocortisone phonophoresis. *Soobschch. Akad. Nauk. Gruz. S.S.R.* 1971; 63:237–240.

36. Griffin, J. E., Touchstone, J. C., Effects of ultrasonic frequency on phonophoresis of cortisol into swine tissues. *Am. J. Phys. Med.* 1972; 51:62.

37. Griffin, J. E., Touchstone, J. S., Ultrasonic movement of cortisol into pig tissue. I. Movement into skeletal muscle. *Am. J. Phys. Med.* 1963; 42:77–85.

38. Griffin, J. E., Touchstone, J. S., Ultrasonic movement of cortisol into pig tissue. II. Movement into paravertebral nerve. *Am. J. Phys. Med.* 1965; 44:20–25.

39. Griffin, J. E., Touchstone, J. C., Low-intensity phonophoresis of cortisol in swine. *Phys. Ther.* 1968; 48(12):1336–1344.

40. Pratzel, H., Dittrich, P., Kukovetz, W., Spontaneous and forced cutaneous absorption of indomethacin in pigs and humans. *J. Rheumatol.* 1986; 13:1122–1125.

41. Kremkau, F. W., Ultrasonic treatment of experimental animal tumors. *Br. J. Cancer.* 1982; 45(Suppl. 5):226–232.

42. Tachibana, K., Tachibana, S., Transdermal delivery of insulin by ultrasonic vibration. *J. Pharm. Pharmacol.* 1991; 43:270–271.

43. Tachibana, K., Tachibana, S., Use of ultrasound to enhance the local anesthetic effect of topically applied aqueous lidocaine. *Anesthesiology* 1993; 78:1091–1096.

44. Kost, J., Levy, D., Langer, R., *Ultrasound Effect on Transdermal Drug Delivery.* Controlled Release Society, Norfolk, VA, 1986: 177–178.

45. Kost, J., Levy, D., Langer, R., *Ultrasound as a Transdermal Enhancer,* 2nd ed., Marcel Dekker, New York, 1989: 595–601.

46. Levy, D., Kost, J., Mashulam, Y., Langer, R., Effect of ultrasound on transdermal drug delivery to rats and guinea pigs. *J. Clin. Invest.* 1989; 83:2074–2078.

47. Miyazaki, S., Mizuoka, H., Oda, M., Takada, M., External control of drug release and penetration: enhancement of the transdermal absorption of indomethacin by ultrasound irradiation. *J. Pharm. Pharmacol.* 1991; 43:115–116.

48. Bommannan, D., Okuyama, H., Stauffer, P., Guy, R. H., Sonophoresis. I: The use of high-frequency ultrasound to enhance transdermal drug delivery. *Pharm. Res.* 1992; 9:559–564.

49. Bommannan, D., Menon, G. K., Okuyama, H., Elias, P. M., Guy, R. H., Sonophoresis. II: Examination of the mechanisms of ultrasound-enhanced transdermal drug delivery. *Pharm. Res.* 1992; 9:1043–1047.

50. Mitragotri, S., Blankschtein, D., Langer, R., Ultrasound-mediated transdermal protein delivery. *Science* 1995; 269:850–853.

51. Nanavaty, M., Brucks, R., Grimes, H., Siegel, F. P. *An ATR-FTIR Approach to Study the Effect of Ultrasound on Human Skin.* Controlled Release Society, Chicago, 1989: 310–311.

52. Mitragotri, S., Edwards, D., Blankschtein, D., and Langer, R., A mechanistic study of ultrasonically-enhanced transdermal drug delivery, *J. Pharm. Sci.* 1995; 84:697–706.

53. Goodman, M., Barry, B. W., Action of skin permeation enhancers azone, oleic acid and decylmethyl sulphoxide: permeation and DSC studies. *J. Pharm. Pharmacol.* 1986; 38(Suppl.):71.

54. Kost, J., Machluf, M., Langer, R., *Experimental Approaches to Elucidate the Mechanism of Ultrasonically Enhanced Transdermal Drug Delivery.* Controlled Release Society, Reno, NV, 1990: 29–30.

55. Mortimer, A. J., Trollope, B. J., Villneuve, E. J., Roy, O. Z., Ultrasound-enhanced diffusion through isolated frog skin. *Ultrasonics* 1988; 26:348–351.

56. Mortimer, A. J., Maclean, J. A., A dosimeter for ultrasonic cavitation. *J. Ultrasound Med.* 1986; 5(Suppl.):137.

57. Simonin, J.-P., On the mechanisms of in vitro and in vivo phonophoresis, *J. Controlled Release* 1995; 33:125–141.

58. Howkins, S. D., Diffusion rates and the effect of ultrasound. *Ultrasonics* 1969; 8:129–130.

59. Fogler, S., Lund, K., Acoustically augmented diffusional transport. *J. Acoust. Soc. Am.* 1973; 53:59–64.

60. Nyborg, W. L., *Acoustic Streaming.* Academic Press, New York, 1965: 265–332.

61. Kost, J., Liu, L.-S., Ferreira, J., Langer, R., Enhanced protein blotting from PhastGel media to membranes by irradiation of low-intensity ultrasound. *Anal. Biochem.* 1994; 216:27–32.

62. Lenart, I., Auslander, D., The effect of ultrasound on diffusion through membranes. *Ultrasonics* 1980; 18:216–218.

63. Julian, T. N., Zentner, G. M., Ultrasonically mediated solute permeation through polymer barriers. *J. Pharm. Pharmacol.* 1986; 38:871–877.

64. Julian, T. N., Zentner, G. M., Mechanism for ultrasonically enhanced transmembrane solute permeation. *J. Controlled Release* 1990; 12:77–85.

65. Kost, J., Leong, K., Langer, R., Ultrasound-enhanced polymer degradation and release of incorporated substances. *Proc. Natl. Acad. Sci. U.S.A.* 1989; 86:7663–7666.

66. Kost, J., Liu, L.-S., Gabelnick, H., Langer, R., Ultrasound as a potential trigger to terminate the activity of contraceptive delivery implants. *J. Controlled Release* 1994; 30:77–81.

67. Liu, L.-S., Kost, J., D'Emanuele, A., Langer, R., Experimental approach to elucidate the mechanism of ultrasound-enhanced polymer erosion and release of incorporated substances. *Macromolecules* 1992; 25:123–128.

68. D'Emanuele, A., Kost, J., Hill, J., Langer, R., An investigation of the effect of ultrasound on degradable polyanhydride matrices. *Macromolecules* 1992; 25:511–515.

Index

Index